Fundamentals of Sound with Applications to Speech and Hearing

Fundamentals of Sound with Applications to Speech and Hearing

---

William J. Mullin
University of Massachusetts Amherst
William J. Gerace
University of Massachusetts Amherst
Jose P. Mestre
University of Massachusetts Amherst
Shelley L. Velleman
University of Massachusetts Amherst

Boston   New York   San Francisco
Mexico City   Montreal   Toronto   London   Madrid   Munich   Paris
Hong Kong   Singapore   Tokyo   Cape Town   Sydney

Executive Editor & Publisher: Stephen D. Dragin
Editorial Assistant: Barbara Strickland
Marketing Manager: Tara Whorf
Editorial Production Service: Chestnut Hill Enterprises, Inc.
Composition Buyer: Linda Cox
Manufacturing Buyer: Andrew Turso
Cover Administrator: Kristina Mose-Libon
Electronic Composition: Publishers' Design and Production Services, Inc.

For related titles and support materials, visit our online catalog at www.ablongman.com.

Between the time Website information is gathered and then published, it is not unusual for some sites to have closed. Also, the transcription of URLs can result in unintended typographical errors. The publisher would appreciate notification where these errors occur so that they may be corrected in subsequent editions.

Library of Congress Cataloging-in-Publication Data

Fundamentals of sound with applications to speech and hearing / by W.J. Mullin . . . [et al.].
    p. cm
   Includes index.
   ISBN 0-205-37087-X
   1. Sound. 2. Speech. 3. Hearing. I. Title: Fundamentals of sound. II. Mullin, William J.
QC225.15 .F86 2003
534—dc21   2002026172

Printed in the United States of America

10   9   8   7   6   5   4   3   2   1   08   07   06   05   04   03   02

To our families

Contents

Preface

Students and workers from several fields, such as communication studies, communication disorders, linguistics, and health sciences, are interested in the mechanisms of speech and hearing. The physics of sound is basic to the understanding of how we communicate, but students in these fields often have not taken a general physics course and may not possess the background for attaining a deep understanding within their own area of study. This book is meant to provide the background in the physics of sound, at a level appropriate for undergraduate non-physical-science majors, for further study of speech and hearing.

Our students, while bright and hardworking, often do not have strong backgrounds in science and mathematics. They need material that provides qualitative insight into the nature of sound. We provide that in this book by the frequent use of graphical illustrations. Animations are included on an associated Web site. We use math at the level of algebra because without that, understanding is simply too imprecise to be able to develop the ideas at a level to promote conceptual understanding. However, the math is always accompanied by a thorough verbal interpretation. There is no necessity for the reader to have had previous experience in physics or a physics course.

The Physics Department at the University of Massachusetts introduced a course in the physics of sound, with applications to speech and hearing, in the early 1970s. Since then, almost every major in the Communications Disorders Department at the university has taken this course as a prerequisite to their speech and hearing science courses. A substantial percentage of the students in the course were from other majors as well, and have taken the course to satisfy departmental or general education science requirements, or sometimes for general interest. The three of the authors of this book who are in the Physics Department have been involved at one time or another in teaching and writing classnotes for the course, which have developed into this book. The fourth coauthor (SLV) has taught the subsequent speech science course in the Communication Disorders Department.

Preferences for notation and terms sometimes differ between communication sciences and physics. While we have tried to strike a compromise between the two disciplines, we have often favored the communication science notation because of the expected readership. For example, physicists prefer to call a fundamental frequency f_1, whereas communication scientists use f_0, and we conform to the latter usage. Physicists use f_n for the nth harmonic, whereas that notation would not be sensible when the counting begins with 0; thus, we denote the nth harmonic simply as nf_0. When resonance occurs, the physicists tend to call *both* the source and resonator component frequencies "fundamental," "harmonics," and "overtones." The communication sciences carefully distinguish the source and resonator and denote the resonator modes by "lowest natural resonant frequency (LNRF)," "higher natural resonant frequencies," and "formants." The latter notational approach may help the reader avoid confusion in learning about the speech mechanism (Chapter 8), so we introduce the distinction in Chapter 4, Resonance.

The Web site associated with the book contains supplementary material that the reader should find useful. Sound is a wave, and as such it is a dynamic quantity. Frozen graphics are inadequate to convey understanding without a struggle by the reader. For this reason, the Web site contains animations that show such situations much more clearly. The Web site also contains a tutorial that can be used to help the reader with some of the harder concepts or as a self-test. The tutorial includes many multiple-choice questions involving every concept in the book. Users click on answers; when they choose incorrect answers, they receive hints and can retry. The official correct answer and a detailed explanation are available at a click. Throughout the book are scattered problems or questions denoted by "Answer This." The reader is meant to work independently on these problems and then look up the answers on the Web site. Any reference to Web-related material is signaled by an icon ✸ in the margins of the book. Further exercises not contained in the Web tutorial are included at the end of each chapter.

Acknowledgments

We would like to thank William Leonard, Uma Balakrishnan, Richard Freyman, Peter Chikov, and Courtney Bolser for their help in preparing the manuscript. In addition, we thank the following reviewers for their insightful comments: Craig A. Champlin, University of Texas at Austin; Daniel C. Halling, James Madison University; and Virginia A. Hinton, University of North Carolina-Greensboro.

1

Introduction to Waves

You want to tell your friend about the great physics book you have just read. You search your brain for the right words and you speak them; you hear yourself speaking and make sure the words that correctly express your ideas are coming from your mouth. All this occurs rather automatically. Your friend hears the words, and they trigger a set of thoughts in her mind. You have transferred your ideas to her. She probably will respond with comments. This oral communication takes place every day among billions of people, but it is an amazingly complicated process.

Communication, in general, consists of three parts: generation, propagation, and reception. In verbal communication, generation refers to speech; propagation refers to the movement of sound waves in space from speaker to hearer; and reception refers to the process of hearing. The phrase "speech chain" refers to the events linking the speaker's brain with the listener's brain; this chain includes generation of speech, feedback link to the speaker, propagation of sound waves, reception by the listener, and transmission of information from the hearing mechanism to the brain. Clearly, the processes necessary involve strong interactions among the physical, physiological, and psychological aspects of the world and our bodies. A thorough study of all of these elements as they relate to spoken communication is called psychoacoustics. This text, while it will mention the necessary aspects of physiology and psychology, will emphasize the physics of speech and hearing.

What is sound? How does it travel from speaker to hearer? One thing that we will quickly learn is that sound needs a **medium** in which to propagate. Sound can propagate in media such as air, water, rocks, and so on that have special properties, such as elasticity, that allow it to travel. We will be concerned mainly with studying propagation of sound in air. When you hear sound, what actually propagates through the air

is pressure disturbances. These pressure disturbances can be described in terms of **wave** phenomena. Thus, for our purposes **sound is a wave in air**. The pressure disturbances travel as a wave—they constitute the wave—traveling through the medium of air. When the pressure disturbance reaches your ear, you hear sound. Obviously, we need to investigate more fully what are waves, what is meant by the term "pressure disturbance," and how the ear detects a sound.

There are many instances of waves in nature. We are all familiar with water waves, for example. Most of us have shaken a rope to make an S-like curve move along it. Plucking a violin or guitar string makes the string vibrate as a wave. All these waves, and nearly any other example of a wave that you can think of, require some medium for propagation. Water waves require water to propagate; waves on a string or rope require the string or rope as medium. (The major exception is electromagnetic waves, including light waves, radio or TV waves, and X rays, which do not require a medium for propagation. Unlike sound waves, light can propagate through a complete vacuum.)

The word "wave" can refer to many different physical phenomena: water waves, sound waves, and so on. However, we can make an abstraction of the concept of wave that contains the properties common to *all* types of waves. Once we have done this, we can apply these general concepts to describe sound propagation in particular. Unlike, say, water waves, we cannot see sound waves, except indirectly through electronic equipment, so it is easier to use examples that one can actually see.

In this chapter, we introduce the basic concepts of wave motion, including the general categories of waves such as transverse waves, longitudinal waves, sinusoidal waves, and impulsive waves. We define many terms that are used to describe waves, such as

---

❀ indicates that the student can find related material on the Web site.

frequency and wavelength, and investigate phenomena that involve wave interactions, such as interference and reflection. We discuss the properties of a medium that are necessary for waves to propagate and describe how waves travel in air. Finally, we apply this information to sound waves.

You might do the following experiment to prepare for reading the next sections. Take a shallow pan of water—the wider the pan the better. Dip your finger in the water in the middle of the pan; note that circles move away from where your finger touched the water. The circles are made of regions where the water is deeper or shallower than normal. These circles make up a wave. However, there is a peculiarity that you may not have noticed before. If you float a small cork in the water and repeat the finger dipping, the cork mainly moves up and down, while the circles (the waves) spread out away from the center. The water is *not* flowing from the center to the sides; any individual element of water is simply moving up and down like the cork; and yet the wave is spreading out with a certain speed. The wave disturbance is being transferred from one element of water to a neighboring one, and then to the next, and so on. Note also that the speed with which the circles move is always the same. Even if you dip your finger in the water more quickly or more often, the speed with which the waves spread does not change. Further, you should notice that when one of your waves reaches the edge of the pan, it bounces off and starts back towards the center. If waves are still spreading outward, the incoming waves and outgoing waves seem to pass through one another.

The pan of water is sometimes called a ripple tank and is very useful for illustrating properties of waves. We will refer to it several time in what follows, and will also use an even easier example of waves on a string. Perhaps thinking about the ripple tank experiment will help you make more sense out of the following sections.

1-A. Types of Waves

Crudely defined, a wave is a disturbance traveling in an elastic medium. When one region of the material is disturbed from equilibrium, it is pulled toward its normal location. (In a water wave, if the water is above normal height, gravity pulls it down; if it is below, it gets pushed back up by the surrounding water.) Meanwhile, the disturbance in the original position in turn disturbs the material in the neighboring regions so that the wave moves to the next region. In the water wave you made in the pan of water, the cir-

cles expand as one region disturbs the next region of larger radius. Waves can be described as either transverse or longitudinal depending on the motion of the medium through which the wave moves.

Transverse waves are waves in which the particles in the medium move perpendicular to the direction in which the wave travels. Examples of transverse waves are water waves, waves on strings, and the "wave" that fans make at a sporting event. (The latter are not really waves since the medium—the fans—is not really elastic, but the motion has a lot in common with a true wave.) The wave in the ripple tank moves outward in an expanding circle, but the water itself moves only up and down, at right angles to the wave direction.

Longitudinal waves are waves in which the particles in the medium move parallel to the direction in which the wave itself travels. Examples of longitudinal waves are sound waves and waves traveling along the coiled toy known as a Slinky. Hang a Slinky downward, and give it a quick shake in the up-down direction. A crowding of the coils moves downward. The crowding is the wave; an individual coil just moves down and up quickly as the wave goes by. That medium motion is in the vertical direction, just as is the wave itself, which is going down.

Suppose we consider a wave on a very long rope or string when someone is shaking the end of the rope smoothly up and down so that waves move away regularly. With the right motion, the person will be making what is called a sinusoidal wave. The motion of the medium is up and down (transverse), while the waves move horizontally along the rope. Figure 1-1 ✿ shows an "animation" of a transverse sinusoidal wave on a rope. (The term "sinusoidal" will be discussed below.) Note that while the crests (peaks) of the wave move to the right, each bit of the string (for example, the one where the black dot is situated) moves up and down in a direction perpendicular (transverse) to the direction in which the wave travels.

Figure 1-2 ✿ shows an "animation" of a longitudinal sinusoidal wave. Think of a wave on a Slinky with the spring loops represented by the dots or a sound wave where the dots represent molecules of air. In this wave, a wave crest is any dense grouping of dots, which moves to the right. Try to follow such a grouping with your finger as you move down the page; notice that the dense region moves to the right. However, any one dot (such as the one with the circle around it) has the motion of the medium; that is, it moves left and right alternately. The motion of the medium is along the direction in which the wave is

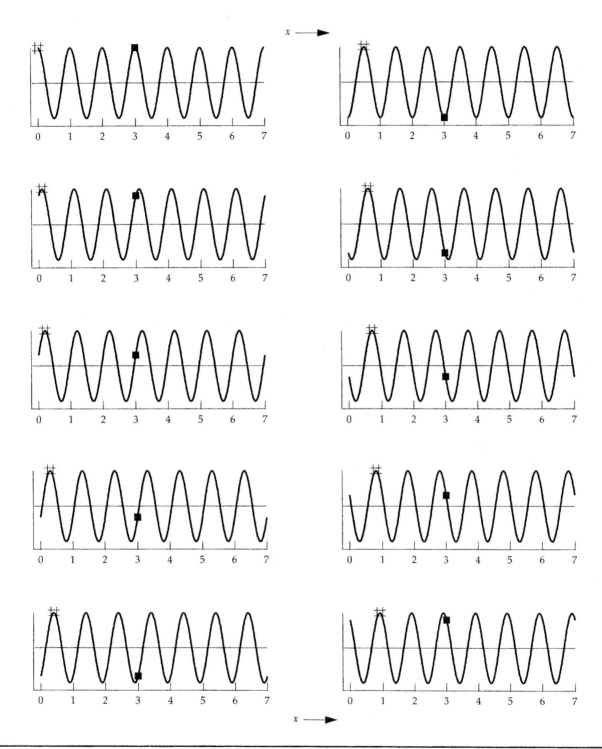

FIGURE 1-1   Transverse wave. Examine this series by moving down the first column from the top; then move to the top of the second column and go down again. Motion then repeats from the top. The medium moves only up and down, while the wave moves to the right. Note that the small black square moving with the medium always stays at $x = 3$, but it goes up and down as the wave goes by. Follow the wave motion by examining the same crest in each figure. The crest at the left end of the first figure (marked #) is initially at $x = 0$, while at the top of the second column it is at $x = 0.5$, and it finally has moved almost to $x = 1$ in the last figure. (This effect is much easier to see in the animation on the Web site associated with this book. There you can view multiple cycles.)

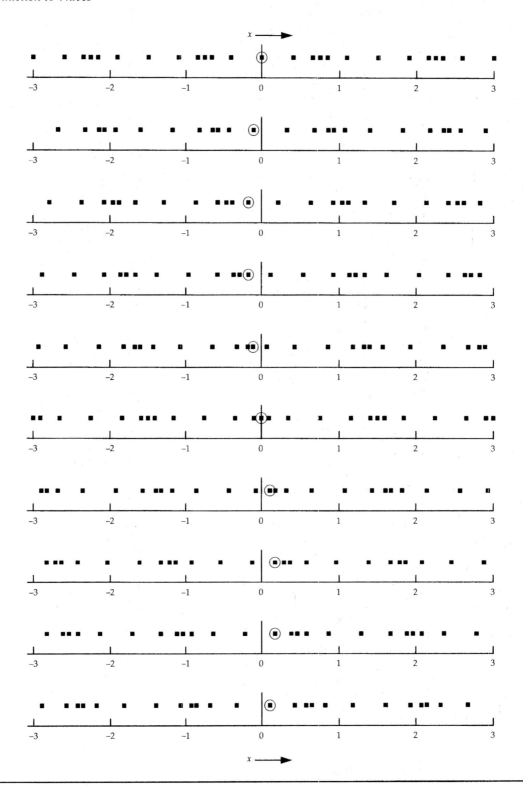

FIGURE 1-2   Longitudinal wave. Move from top to bottom, after which the motion starts over at the top. The medium motion is shown by the circled dot. It moves back and forth around $x = 0$, but makes no net progress. The wave motion is followed by noting how a density crest (a group of particles close together) moves from left to right. Note that the density crest near $x = -0.8$ at the top moves to the right until it includes the circled dot at $x = 0$ in picture 6 and then moves on past to about $x = 0.6$ in the bottom picture. (The medium and wave motion are easier to see in the animation on the Web site associated with this book. There you can watch multiple cycles.)

traveling, and that is why this type of wave is called longitudinal.

Waves may also be classified as **traveling** or **standing** waves. The waves in Figures 1-1 and 1-2 are traveling waves; any wave crest can be seen to be traveling to the right in each figure. Of course, a wave crest might equally well travel to the left. The wave you made in the pan of water was a traveling wave moving outward. The other classification, standing waves, will be explained in Chapter 2.

1-B. Wave Shapes

Both transverse and longitudinal waves come in several possible forms. What, for example, is the difference in the sound waves produced by an exploding balloon and those produced by a musical instrument playing a single sustained note? A partial answer is that the first is impulsive and the second oscillatory. **Impulsive waves shapes** are made up of a single burst of one or several pulses. For example, a bang noise, such as clapping your hands, has an impulsive wave shape. Moving your hand up and down once on the end of a taut rope that is tied to a tree will produce an impulsive wave. **Oscillatory wave shapes** always have a definite repeating pattern. The pattern can be complicated, but it is repeated over and over.

Sinusoidal wave shapes are oscillatory waves that have a special simple shape like a mathematical sine or cosine curve. This type of wave is easily recognized by its smooth undulating shape. A vibrating tuning fork can give rise to a sinusoidal sound wave. A musical instrument usually produces an oscillatory wave that is not sinusoidal. Sinusoidal waves are useful for studying the properties of standing waves (discussed later). Figure 1-3 shows examples of possible wave forms: (a) two impulsive waves, (b) a sinusoidal wave, and (c) an oscillatory wave that is *not* sinusoidal.

1-C. Propagation Velocity and Medium Velocity

When a person dips her finger in the water in the water-in-a-pan experiment, the circular waves spread out at a certain speed. We want to investigate this speed and what determines it. When you drive a car you determine speed by looking at the speedometer. But you could also figure out an average speed by dividing the number of miles you traveled by the time you needed to drive that distance (miles per hour). Consider a pulse wave on a string. The **propagation**

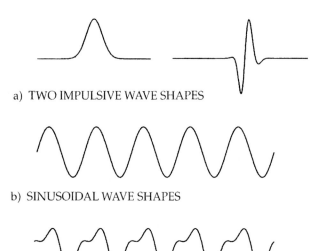

a) TWO IMPULSIVE WAVE SHAPES

b) SINUSOIDAL WAVE SHAPES

c) OSCILLATORY WAVE THAT IS NOT SINUSOIDAL

FIGURE 1-3 (a) Impulsive waves are made up of one or a few nonrepeating pulses. (b) A sinusoidal wave has the smooth repeating shape shown, which is the plot of the sine or cosine curve in mathematics. (c) Not all oscillatory waves are sinusoidal. This one has a repeating shape, and so is oscillatory, but it does not have the sinusoidal shape shown in (b).

velocity (or **wave velocity**) of a pulse on a string is the speed at which the pulse moves along on the string. Since **speed is distance divided by time**, we can find the propagation speed of a pulse by measuring how far a particular point on the pulse traveled—call it D—and the time it took it to travel this distance—call it T—and computing D/T. Figure 1-4 shows this procedure applied to an impulsive wave. The propagation velocity of sound (the speed of sound) in air is approximately 760 miles per hour, more than 10 times the speed limit for a car on a highway.

In the ripple tank, there is another speed you could determine if you had a cork floating in the water. This is the speed with which the cork bobs up or down. We distinguish this velocity from that of the circular wave moving outward and call it the **medium velocity**. The direction of this velocity keeps changing from up to down and back again as the wave passes.

The **medium velocity** is the speed with which a point of the medium moves as the wave passes that point. Note that in the case of a pulse moving along a string, any given point on the string has 0 speed before the wave arrives. It picks up speed as it moves up,

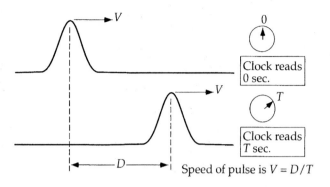

FIGURE 1-4 The propagation velocity, or wave velocity, of a pulse wave is determined by dividing the distance traveled, D, by the time, T, needed to travel this distance.

stops (0 speed again) when the peak of the pulse coincides with the point, and then picks up speed again as it comes back down. For an animated view of this see the answer to Question 5 on the Web tutorial ✸

Example: Your car travels at a steady speed and goes 100 miles in 4 hours. What is its velocity?

Solution: Divide distance (100 mi) by time (4 hr) to find the velocity.

$$V = D/T = 100 \text{ mi}/4 \text{ hr} = 25 \text{ mph}$$

where mph means miles per hour.

Example: Suppose that a pulse wave travels 5 meters along a string in 2 seconds. What is the propagation velocity v?

Solution: $v = \dfrac{5 \text{ meters}}{2 \text{ seconds}} = 2.5 \text{ m/s}$

(m/s is read meters per second).

Note: Appendix A provides an introduction to the metric system of units.

Example: A cork bobs up and back down as a water wave goes by. It rises to a height of 0.2 m in 0.5 s and then drops down again after the wave has passed. What was its average medium velocity on the way up?

Solution: $v = 0.2 \text{ m}/0.5 \text{ s} = 0.4 \text{ m/s}$.

✸ ANSWER THIS

(Answers and discussions of all the Answer-This questions can be found on the text Web site. Additional such questions will be found there as well.)

- If a very small ribbon is glued at a point on a rubber rope and an impulsive wave is sent along the rope from left to right, what will happen to the ribbon?

  a) It will move with the medium velocity.

  b) It will travel along the rope from left to right.

  c) It will not move.

  d) It will move with the wave velocity.

  e) It will travel at 760 mph.

1-D. Sinusoidal Waves: More Terminology

Let's consider a sinusoidal wave on a string in order to introduce some other useful definitions. Figure 1-5 shows five different snapshots of a string at five equally spaced intervals of time; the wave on this string is sinusoidal. There are five properties of waves: wavelength, cycle, period, amplitude, and frequency. Some are interrelated. We will define them and then give examples.

- The **wavelength** is the distance from one peak of the wave to the next adjacent peak (or equivalently, the distance between two adjacent troughs—the low points of the waves). The wavelength measures the length of the wave segment that keeps repeating itself. The symbol given to wavelength is the Greek letter λ (lambda). Wavelength has the dimensions of length (feet, inches, meters, etc.).

  The point on the string labeled B in Figure 1-5 oscillates up and down with the medium velocity, which was discussed earlier. A **cycle** is a complete round trip of point B from its original position, up, down all the way to its lowest position, and back up to its original position. (Two cycles means two round trips, three cycles is three round trips, and so on.)

- The **displacement** is the distance that point B (or other point) is moved from its normal nonvibrating position.

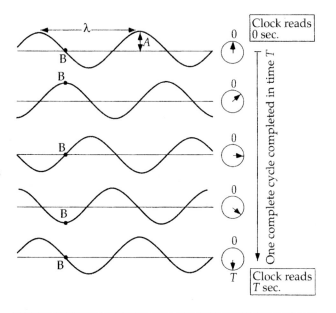

Clock reads 0 sec.

One complete cycle completed in time T

Clock reads T sec.

FIGURE 1-5   A sinusoidal wave shown at successive times. A crest or peak moves to the right at the wave velocity. A point of the medium, B, moves up and down as the wave passes through a full cycle. The wavelength is denoted by λ, and one full period T elapses during this cycle.

- The **amplitude** is the maximum distance that point B is displaced from its normal nonvibrating position. We use the capital letter A to denote the amplitude. Amplitude is the maximum value of the displacement.
- The **period** is the time required to complete one cycle (time per cycle) and is denoted by the letter T. Period is measured in units of time, usually seconds.
- The **frequency**, which we denote by the letter f, is the number of **cycles per second** of time. The unit cycles per second is usually shortened to **Hertz**—that is, two cycles per second is written 2 Hertz or 2 Hz.

Suppose that the point B makes two complete cycles in one second. Then the frequency would be 2 cycles per second (2 Hz). If point B made five cycles in two seconds, the frequency would be 2.5 cycles per second (2.5 Hz). Note that you get the frequency by dividing the total number of cycles by the time it took to complete them.

Example: Suppose a water wave has a crest that travels 5 meters in 2 seconds. (A meter is about 39 inches. See Appendix A for an introduction to the metric system of units.) A boat floating in the water drops 1 meter below normal and rises 1 meter above normal when the wave passes. The boat takes 1 second to go from its lowest position to its highest. What is the wave velocity, amplitude, period, and frequency? Can you also figure out the wavelength?

Solution: You can pretend the boat is point B in Figure 1-5. The propagation or wave velocity is the distance the wave crest moves divided by the time it takes to move that distance or 5 m/2 s = 2.5 m/s. The amplitude is the distance from normal level to highest, or 1 meter (not the 2 meters from lowest point to highest). The period of the wave is the time for a complete cycle—in other words, the time to go from lowest point to highest and back down to lowest, which is 2 seconds. If the boat takes 2 seconds to do one cycle, it must be doing only 1/2 cycle per second. Thus the frequency is 0.5 Hz.

Finding the wavelength is a bit trickier: The boat (point B in Figure 1-5) is at normal height in the first part of the figure. Note a crest at the left of it. While the boat moves through one complete cycle, from top figure element to bottom element, this crest moves to the right exactly one wavelength. Thus, the **wavelength is the distance a wave moves in one period**. The distance traveled is velocity times time, $D = v \times T$, or in this case $\lambda = v \times T = 2.5 \text{ m/s} \times 2 \text{ s} = 5 \text{ m}$.

While studying the example, you may have noticed that there is a very simple relationship between the period and the frequency. Suppose that point B is oscillating with a frequency of 1/2 Hz. This means that it takes 2 seconds to complete one cycle, so the period is 2 seconds. If instead, point B were to oscillate with a frequency of 3 cycles per second, it would take 1/3 second to make one cycle, so the period would be 1/3 second. Notice the pattern: You get the period by taking the reciprocal of the frequency. Conversely, you can get the frequency by taking the reciprocal of the period. Expressed in math notation, we have:

$$T = \frac{1}{f} \quad \text{or} \quad f = \frac{1}{T}.$$

Summary of Definitions

Wave (or **propagation**) **velocity**: The speed with which a crest or any other part of the wave moves in the direction of the wave.

Medium velocity: The speed with which any portion of the medium's material moves as a wave goes by. This motion is either perpendicular to the wave velocity in a transverse wave or along it in a longitudinal wave.

Wavelength: The distance between two corresponding points on the wave (i.e., the distance for which the wave repeats). Symbol: λ.

Cycle: One complete oscillation, or one complete round trip of a point in the medium.

Period: The time it takes to complete one cycle. Symbol: T.

Frequency: The number of cycles per second (often denoted cps, but Hz is preferred). Symbol: f.

Displacement: Distance of a point from its equilibrium position (the position when there is no wave).

Amplitude: Maximum displacement of the string. Symbol: A.

❈ ANSWER THIS

- A 15-foot-long rubber rope is tied to the wall. It takes an impulsive wave 3 seconds to travel down the rope, reflect, and come back to where it started. What is the wave velocity in feet per second (ft/s)?

  a) 5 ft/s

  b) 10 ft/s

  c) 15 ft/s

  d) 20 ft/s

  e) none of these

- A mass on a spring bobs down and back up 40 times in 10 seconds. What is its frequency in Hertz? 4

1-E. Oscillating Things and Sinusoidal Waves

If we center our attention on a piece of the medium as a wave passes, such as Point B of Figure 1-5, we see that it simply oscillates up and down with the medium motion. This could be a cork on a ripple tank, or a knot on a vibrating string. The motion of this object is similar to that of other things that oscillate, such as the pendulum of a clock or a weight on a spring. Let us plot the motion of such a vibrating object, but now versus time rather than position. Figure 1-6 shows two oscillating systems, a simple pendulum and a block attached to a spring. However, the object could as well be Point B in Figure 1-5.

In both cases, one can use a sinusoidal wave shape to describe the displacement of the oscillating object. The wave shape drawn on the graph in Figure 1-6 describes how the displacement changes with time. At time 0, the displacements for both systems are 0 because the positions of both the block and the pendulum are the equilibrium positions that both systems would have if there were no oscillations. At 1 second and 3 seconds, the pendulum and the block are farthest from their equilibrium positions. At time 2 seconds, the displacements of both systems are 0 since both are back to the equilibrium position. At 1 second, the displacement is maximum, but notice that it is plotted below the horizontal line on the graph to denote negative displacement. (A positive displacement measures distance to one side of equilibrium and a negative displacement measures distance to the

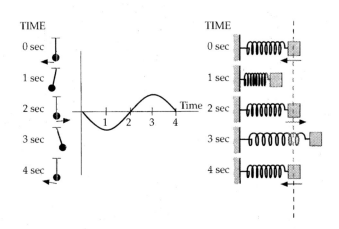

FIGURE 1-6 A plot of the motion of two oscillating things, a pendulum and a mass on a spring. The vertical axis is the displacement of the object from its equilibrium position, which is straight down for the pendulum and at the dotted line for the mass on the spring. A displacement of either object to the right is plotted above the horizontal time axis, and to the left below the horizontal axis. Thus one can tell where the object is at any time. The resulting wave form is sinusoidal.

other side of equilibrium). At 4 seconds, both systems are again at their equilibrium positions. Thus, note that plotting the displacement as time goes by gives a sinusoidal wave shape that represents the motion of *both* systems. Such a plot could also be used to show the vertical displacement of Point B in Figure 1-5 versus time. Note that the plot shown in Figure 1-6 gives exactly one cycle of the motion, and that the time from beginning to end is one period.

1-F. Application of the Concept of Waves to Sound

A **tuning fork** is a useful tool to explore how one might apply waves to describe sound. We know two facts:

- A medium (air) is necessary for sound to propagate to us so that we can hear it.
- There seems to be a connection between vibrations and sound.

When we strike a tuning fork, the prongs move sinusoidally. The series of five pictures in Figure 1-7 depicts one cycle of the fork as the prongs move in time through one complete round trip. The frequency with which the prongs vibrate is the number of these cycles that take place in one second. Recall that frequency is measured in cycles per second, or Hertz (Hz). For example, a particular tuning fork might vibrate at a frequency of 1000 cycles per second, or 1000 Hertz.

Note the following observations regarding tuning forks.

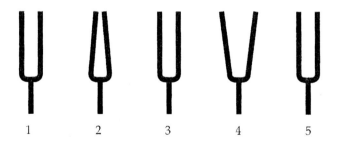

1   2   3   4   5

FIGURE 1-7   A vibrating tuning fork as it undergoes a complete cycle. Each successive picture represents a position at a slightly later time than the preceding one.

- A sinusoidal wave shape plot, as in Figure 1-6, can be used to describe the displacement of the prongs. This wave shape would have a specific frequency, which could be determined by counting the number of oscillations of the prongs in one second.
- Different tuning forks that vibrate at different frequencies sound different. Our auditory system allows us to distinguish different frequencies. This sensation is called **pitch**. The greater the frequency of vibrations, the higher the pitch. Notice that a physical characteristic, namely the frequency of vibrations, gets perceived as a physiological and psychological characteristic, namely pitch.
- If we strike the tuning fork harder, thereby giving it a larger amplitude, we perceive it as sounding louder. (You can't make the fork vibrate at a different frequency by hitting it harder—it always vibrates at the same frequency, producing a sound called a **pure tone**). We associate the physical characteristic of amplitude with the perception called **loudness**.

Although this example has provided some important observations, we still don't know what the tuning fork does to the air to produce the waves we perceive as sound. A model to explain what happens when the tuning fork vibrates is needed. We must now turn to basic elements of molecular theory and observe that air consists of a large number of loosely packed **molecules**. These molecules constantly move around and bump into one another. If undisturbed, this moving and bumping takes place at random.

A few numbers should suitably impress you about the motion of air molecules. First, there are more than 10^{20} molecules in one cubic inch of air (that's a 1 followed by twenty zeros, or 100 billion billion). A typical molecule at room temperature travels at an average speed of 1000 miles an hour and undergoes 10^{10} collisions each second. These air molecules are so loosely packed that they are easily compressed. This is what happens near a vibrating object. As the tuning fork vibrates, it alternately **compresses** and **rarefies** the air in its immediate vicinity. Figure 1-8 shows snapshots of the tuning fork at different times to illustrate the origin of the compressions and rarefactions. The compressions of air are shown as dark regions, while the rarefactions are shown as lighter spaces. The point is that despite the large number of molecules and their random motions, certain disturbances of the air from its normal state will be transmitted through the air.

Since each molecule undergoes a tremendously large number of collisions each second, it is extremely

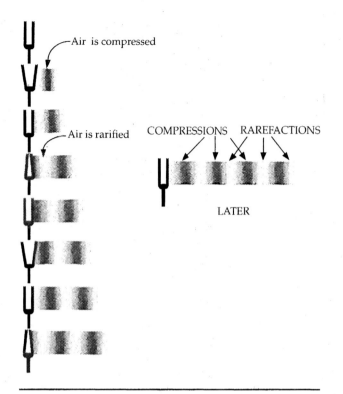

FIGURE 1-8   The tuning fork compresses and rarefies the air as a sound wave is made. The compressions are shown as the darker regions, with rarefactions in between. A sound wave is a series of compressions and rarefactions moving away from the tuning fork.

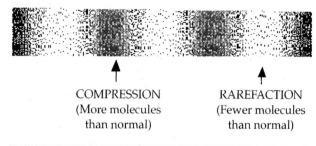

COMPRESSION
(More molecules
than normal)

RAREFACTION
(Fewer molecules
than normal)

FIGURE 1-9   Compressions and rarefactions. Darker regions represent compressions, regions of higher than normal density, while lighter regions represent rarefactions, regions of lower than normal density. Molecules have moved toward the region of a compression, leaving behind rarefactions on either side.

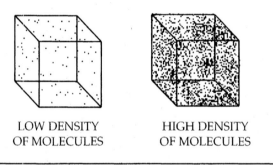

LOW DENSITY
OF MOLECULES

HIGH DENSITY
OF MOLECULES

FIGURE 1-10   A region of low density has fewer molecules in a volume of given size than does a region of high density.

unlikely that your ear is struck by any molecule that was struck by the tuning fork. Rather, your ear is struck by molecules that were struck by molecules that were struck by molecules . . . that were struck by the tuning fork.

Let's look at a more detailed image that models what is happening to the air molecules. If we could see molecules, a representation of the air during the passing of a sound wave might look something like Figure 1-9.

It is now useful to define the concept of **density**, which is the number of molecules in a unit volume. For example, the boxes of air in Figure 1-10 represent the same volume, but in the left box the density is low (because there are relatively few molecules) while in the right box the density is high (because there are many molecules). In summary. rarefactions, are the regions of low density in a sound wave, while compressions are the regions of high density.[*]

Note that where the air is compressed, molecules have moved away from the regions of low density into the regions of high density, and that the medium motion is from right to left or left to right in Figure 1-9, which is along the same direction that the wave is moving. Thus, Figure 1-9 illustrates why **a sound wave is longitudinal.** (See Figure 1-2 for a model showing what is happening in more detail).

Given that a sound wave made by a tuning fork in air has alternating regions of higher-than-average air density and lower-than-average density, we are in a position to apply our wave concept to describe it. A plot of the density of air as a function of position (that is, with density on the vertical axis and position on the horizontal axis) appears in the familiar sinusoidal wave form. Figure 1-11 represents this. Such a sinu-

---

[*] The variation in density is actually very small for a typical sound wave. The density differences in Figures 1-9 and 1-11 are exaggerated for visual clarity.

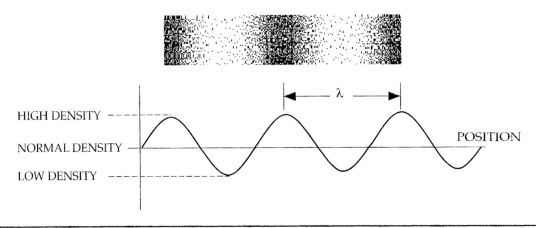

FIGURE 1-11 Plot of density of air molecules versus position. Regions of high density are represented as a displacement above the horizontal axis, while regions of low density are represented as a negative displacement, that is, below the axis.

soidal wave is characteristic of the sound produced by any tuning fork. The resulting sound is known as a **pure tone**. Pure tones are sinusoidal and are perceived differently from the tones produced by musical instruments. Although they are oscillatory, sounds generated by musical instruments are usually more complex than sinusoidal waves.

There is another feature that we might mention in passing: Sound dies out at large distances. The sound wave spreads out spherically from the tuning fork. Think of the analogous thing that happened when you dipped your finger in the ripple tank: Circles of waves spread out from your finger. You may have noticed that their amplitude decreased as the wave got farther from your finger. In the same way, spheres of sound waves expand out from the tuning fork. The density wave becomes so spread out over the surface of the spherical wave as it propagates outward (actually it is wave energy that becomes spread out, as we will see later) that eventually the density change (amplitude) of the wave becomes insignificant at distances far away from the tuning fork.

So far so good. But there seems a problem with our model: Our ear certainly doesn't count molecules, so how does it perceive these density fluctuations? We address this question in Section 1-I. For now, we return to studying waves we can see, like waves on strings, to determine what physical properties of the medium govern the propagation of waves in that medium. This study will ultimately lead us to a property of air that our ears can detect.

1-G. Relationship among v, f, and λ

Envision a traveling wave on a string made by a person waving the end of a rope smoothly up and down. As her arm rises, a crest is created, which moves away; as it falls, a trough is created, and that moves away as well. The arm moves up once more, creating another crest, and the pattern continues. The result is a sinusoidal traveling wave. Snapshots of the rope taken at several time intervals show the propagation of the wave. The four graphs in Figure 1-12 show the rope at four different times separated by intervals of 0.1 second.

The point labeled B on the rope oscillates up and down (at the medium velocity) as we observed before. However, the crest of the wave, tracked at successive times by the dashed line, moves along the rope with the **wave velocity**. See the animation of a traveling transverse wave on the Web site ✱.

This series of snapshots contains all the information about the properties of the wave. For example, the wavelength, λ, is 2 meters. One complete cycle of point B would take 0.4 seconds, so the period, T, is 0.4 seconds. Recall that the frequency can be obtained by taking the reciprocal of the period, thus,

$$f = \frac{1}{T} = \frac{1\text{ cycle}}{0.4\text{ s}} = 2.5\text{ cps} = 2.5\text{ Hz.}$$

The wave crest moves 1.5 meters in 0.3 seconds, so the wave velocity is

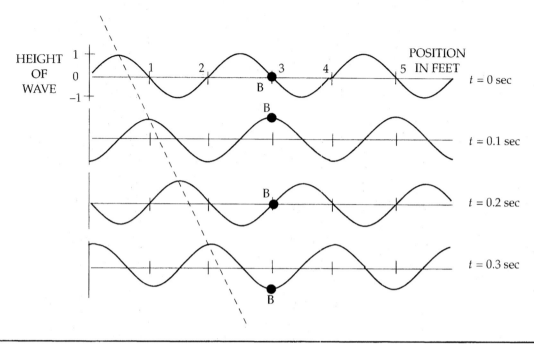

FIGURE 1-12   Wave plot showing the wave height versus position of a transverse traveling wave. The dotted line marks the progress of a single crest of the wave. B marks the motion of the medium.

$$v = \frac{1.5 \text{ m}}{0.3 \text{ s}} = 5 \text{ m/s}.$$

There is another way to find the velocity of a traveling wave. Notice by looking at the snapshots of the propagating wave of Figure 1-12 that in one cycle, the wave travels one wavelength. So the speed of the wave can be found by taking the wavelength and dividing by the time for one cycle. We know that the time of one cycle is just the period, T. So we have:

$$\text{velocity} = \frac{\text{distance}}{\text{time}} = \frac{\text{wavelengh}}{\text{time for one cycle}} = \frac{\lambda}{T}$$

or

$$v = \frac{\lambda}{T},$$

Since $f = \frac{1}{T}$, we also have

$$v = f\lambda.$$

This is an important and useful result. For the example above, recall that $\lambda = 2$ m, $f = 2.5$ Hz, so that,

$v = f\lambda = (2.5 \text{ Hz}) (2 \text{ m}) = 5 \text{ m/s}$, which is the same answer obtained earlier by observing the movement of the crest of the wave. Put simply, if you know the distance between crests (i.e., the wavelength) and you know the number of crests that pass you in some fixed interval of time (i.e., the frequency), then you can compute the speed with which the wave is traveling.

Example: An analogy might make the relation $v = f\lambda$ somewhat clearer. Suppose skiers are moving one by one down a mountain, each at a constant speed of 10 m/s. A starter at the top of the hill determines how often skiers should start down the hill. In the morning, he starts 1 skier every 10 seconds (low frequency), and in the afternoon he starts 1 skier every 5 seconds (high frequency). In which case will the skiers be farther apart? How far apart will they be in each case? The distance between skiers is analogous to the distance between peaks of a wave, the wavelength.

Solution: The skiers will be farther apart when they start off less frequently, namely in the morning. In 10 seconds, the previous skier will have traveled 10 m/s × 10 s = 100 m. In 5 seconds, the previous skier would have traveled 10 m/s × 5 s = 50 m. In terms of $f\lambda = v$:

$$\frac{1 \text{ skier (cycle)}}{10 \text{ s}} \times \frac{100 \text{ m}}{\text{skier (cycle)}} = 0.1 \text{ Hz} \times 100 \text{ m}$$

$$= 10 \text{ m/s}$$

and

$$\frac{1 \text{ skier (cycle)}}{5 \text{ s}} \times \frac{50 \text{ m}}{\text{skier (cycle)}} = 0.2 \text{ Hz} \times 50 \text{ m}$$

$$= 10 \text{ m/s}$$

Thus, the morning skiers are 100 meters apart, and the afternoon skiers are 50 meters apart. Notice that for a given velocity, the higher the frequency, the shorter the wavelength since the product of the two must always equal the velocity, in this case 10 m/s.

In the skier example, the skier's velocity was constant all through the problem as if it were determined by, say, the condition of the snow rather than the skier's ability. In the case of waves, it is indeed the properties of the medium that determine the wave velocity. We examine this next.

1-H. *Wave Velocity and Properties of the Medium*

Let's consider a few of the kinds of materials that can oscillate: a spring, a taut string, a tuning fork, air. The physical property possessed by all these materials is called **elasticity**. **Elastic materials** return to their original shape when bent or disturbed (rubber bands, springs), whereas inelastic materials remain deformed (e.g., a lump of clay).

All material bodies have **mass** and **inertia**. Mass is a measure of the amount of material in a body. The mass of a body depends on the number of the protons, neutrons, and electrons making up the atoms in the body. Mass results in inertia.

Galileo noted early in the seventeenth century that when a body is at rest or in motion, it has a tendency to remain at rest or in motion unless there is a **force** (a push or a pull from something else) that changes that motion. **Inertia** is the tendency of a body

to remain in its present state of motion. If at rest, a body will stay at rest unless there is a force to get it moving; if it is in motion, a force is required to make it move faster or slower. The more mass an object has, the more inertia it has. The more massive a body is (more protons, neutrons, and electrons), the more it resists changes in its state of motion, that is, the more inertia it has.

It is important to distinguish between mass and **weight**. Weight on Earth is the force of Earth's gravity exerted on an object because of its mass. If you jump off the ground, the gravitational attraction Earth has for the mass in your body pulls you back down. However, out in space, far from any massive body, an object would have no weight (because there is no gravity), but it would still have mass (the amount of material it has) and inertia (the resistance to change of its state of motion).

Consider the motion of a block attached to the end of a suspended spring. The five sequential snapshots of Figure 1-13 show the effect of elasticity and inertia. If at rest, the block stays at rest. But, if the spring is initially compressed by some force and then let go as shown in the first picture, the spring's elasticity pushes downward and the gravitational pull of the Earth is also directed down. Together, these forces cause the block to move in a downward direction. However, once it has returned to its original equilibrium position, the block's inertia makes it overshoot the equilibrium position. The block continues to move in a downward direction until the force of elasticity of the spring becomes larger than the force of

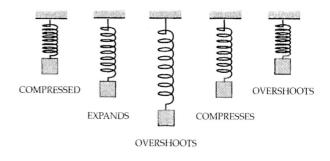

COMPRESSED   OVERSHOOTS

EXPANDS   COMPRESSES

OVERSHOOTS

FIGURE 1-13 Oscillations of a mass on a spring illustrating elasticity and inertia. The initial compression of the spring and gravity pulling on the mass cause the mass to move downward; due to inertia the mass overshoots its equilibrium position, thereby stretching the spring, which eventually pulls the block back upward. It again overshoots and compresses the spring. Oscillations result.

gravity, which causes the block to stop and move back upward. It overshoots again, and so on, giving rise to oscillations. So elasticity and inertia are the ingredients necessary for causing and maintaining waves.

An important question to consider is: Why do oscillations in elastic media eventually stop? The reason all waves eventually die out is friction. (We often consider an ideal world where there is no friction, because it is much harder to build a model that accurately includes friction.) **Friction** is a force caused by the surface roughness of two objects in contact when one object moves relative to the other. The friction on an object always acts to oppose the motion of the object. If you slide a plate across a table, it will come to a stop shortly because friction due to the table slows it down. A vibrating string moving in air feels friction due to air resistance.

Suppose that an elastic material, such as a string of some length and mass, is stretched to a certain tension. Will this material support any combination of wave velocity, frequency, and wavelength that one attempts to send through it? The answer is no. The properties of the medium (type of material, tension, and mass) determine the wave velocity. The wave can have any wavelength or frequency, but the relationship $v = f\lambda$ must always be satisfied. For a given medium, v is fixed, so if f is increased, say by shaking the string more often per second, then the wavelength must decrease so the product $f\lambda$ stays the same. (Recall the example of the skiers, who, when they started more often, were closer together.)

Consider a long spring with one end attached to a wall and the other end held by your hand. If you pull the spring a small amount and send a pulse down the spring (say, by moving your hand up and down once), then the pulse will travel relatively slowly. On the other hand, if you stretch the spring a lot so that it is under greater tension, and the same pulse is sent down the spring, the pulse will travel faster. Increasing the tension increases the elasticity of the medium. The result is that the higher the tension, the higher the wave velocity.

If a heavier (i.e., more massive) spring is used but is stretched to the same tension as some other, less-massive spring, we would find that the pulse would move more slowly in the more-massive spring. The more-massive spring has more inertia. What is actually relevant is the linear mass *density* (the mass per unit length), rather than the mass itself. Thus, the higher the linear mass density, the lower the wave velocity.

To summarize, for waves on springs and ropes, the wave velocity is determined by two physical properties: **tension** and **mass density**. We must now explore similar properties in air that determine the propagation speed (or wave velocity) of sound waves.

❖ ANSWER THIS

- You are given a wave medium with *fixed* elasticity and density. A traveling sinusoidal wave can be created in this medium

  a) of any frequency.

  b) of any wavelength.

  c) of any wave velocity.

  d) both a and b.

  e) a, b, and c.

- If you want to make a wave in a string move very fast (i.e., have a large wave velocity), you can

  a) make the tension in the string large.

  b) use a thin rather than thick string.

  c) jiggle your hand fast to create the wave.

  d) a and b.

  e) a, b, and c.

1-I. Elastic Properties of Air

There are two properties of a gas that are analogous to the tension and linear mass density properties of a spring or rope. Let us first explore what the quantity analogous to tension is in air (clearly it is not tension, since we can't pull on air).

As discussed earlier, air molecules are in motion and move in a random fashion. They are constantly bumping into one another and into the walls of any container filled with air. Molecules are always rebounding from the walls, and this creates a **force** on the wall. (It is somewhat like pushing on a wall by firing rubber bullets from a machine gun at it.) However, the total force on a wall is not quite the quantity we seek; rather, what we are interested in is the pressure. **Pressure** is defined as force per unit area. This quantity is often measured in pounds per square inch, or Newtons per square meter (called Pascals; see Appendix A) in the metric system. Atmospheric pressure (due to the weight of a one inch square column of air in the atmosphere) is about 14.7 pounds per square inch (psi). An example will give an intuitive feel for the physical property we call pressure. Consider a one-pound book placed on your hand. You feel a pressure that is equal to the weight of the book divided by the surface area of your hand. Supposing that your hand has a surface area of about 10 square inches, you would feel a pressure of 1/10 pound per square inch. Now suppose that a pencil is placed point-down on your hand, and the one-pound book is placed on top of the pencil's eraser. You would feel a tremendously large pressure because the same weight, one pound, is now distributed over the very small area that makes up the point of the pencil. Supposing that the area of the pencil point is about 1/1000 square inch, the pressure you would now feel is

$$P = \frac{\text{Force}}{\text{Area}} = \frac{1 \text{ pound}}{1/1000 \text{ square inch}}$$
$$= 1000 \text{ pounds per square inch.}$$

The pressure now would be 10,000 times larger than it was with just the book on top of your hand, and your hand would hurt more than in the first arrangement! Your skin is sensitive to pressure.

As it turns out, it is the pressure of a gas that is the physical quantity analogous to tension in strings. The pressure provides the elasticity of the air. The only difference is that instead of being pulled back to the equilibrium position as with a spring, the molecules of air are pushed back by the pressure. Thus, the higher the gas pressure, the more elastic the air, and the faster sound travels through the gas.

The **volume mass density** (the mass per unit volume) for a gas has the same influence on the speed of sound as linear mass density has on the wave velocity for a string. The volume mass density determines the inertial quality of the air. Thus the larger the volume mass density of a gas, the higher the inertia and (for a fixed average pressure) the slower the speed of the sound wave.

From the study of gases, we know that pressure and density are related to each other. When other things like temperature are held constant, the higher the density, the greater the pressure. We have already observed that there is a correspondence between the wave concept and density fluctuations present during a pure tone sound made by a tuning fork. Because they are related, the pressure must fluctuate in a sinusoidal fashion just like the density. Figure 1-14 de-

picts a sound wave, represented by a pressure wave plotted as a function of position at some fixed time (the diagram represents a snapshot of how the pressure varies in space at a fixed instant in time.) Regions of higher-than-average pressure push molecules toward the regions of lower-than-average pressure, but the inertia of the gas molecules causes an overshoot, and oscillatory waves are the result.

It is the pressure of the gas (force per unit area) that pushes on the ear drum, allowing the ear to perceive sound. Although the ear's functioning will be discussed in Chapter 12, a few introductory remarks are in order. The range of sensitivity of the ear is astounding; we can hear anything from a mosquito flying near our ear to a sonic boom. The ear consists of a chain of pneumatic, mechanical, and hydraulic devices that can compress this extremely large range of sounds to an essentially linear scale of fluid disturbances with surprisingly little distortion. The ear is designed to measure pressure differences, not absolute pressure. The eardrum is a flexible membrane that vibrates with the pressure changes associated with the sound wave. To measure pressure differences, the eardrum is balanced by normal atmospheric pressure from the inner side via the Eustachian tube, as shown in Figure 1-15. Although the Eustachian tube is usually collapsed, when we swallow it opens to atmospheric pressure.

Air pressure is a function of altitude above sea level (and other things like temperature and humidity). If we undergo a large altitude change, as when climbing a mountain, and do not swallow or "pop" our ears as we go along, our ears begin to feel uncomfortable. The eardrum is being pushed from the

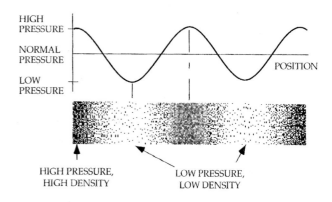

FIGURE 1-14 Relation between density and pressure in a sound wave. Regions of high density have high pressure; low-density regions have low pressure.

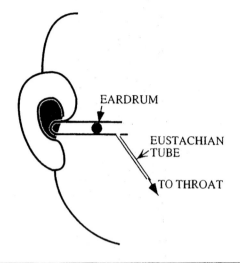

FIGURE 1-15 A schematic diagram of the ear showing how the exterior and interior pressures are maintained nearly equal by the Eustachian tube.

inside by the pressure differences due to the altitude change.

In summary, the wave velocity of a wave on a string depends on the tension and the linear mass density of the string. Analogously, the sound velocity in a gas depends on the pressure and the average volume mass density of the gas. Pressure and tension are called **dynamic** variables because they help propagate waves. Linear mass density and volume mass density are properties of the medium called **inertial** variables because they offer resistance to changes of motion.

❀ANSWER THIS

A hammer hits on the top of a nail with a force of 50 pounds. The nail tip pressing against a piece of wood has an area of 0.01 sq. in. A force of 100 pounds is applied to the top of a uniform cylinder having an area of 1 sq. in. Which exerts the greater pressure on the wood and by how much?

   a) The pressure of the nail is 100 times greater than that of the cylinder.

   b) The pressure of the nail is 50 times greater than that of the cylinder.

   c) The pressure of the cylinder is 2 times greater than that of the nail.

   d) The pressure of the cylinder is 100 times greater than that of the nail.

1-J. Reflection and Transmission of Waves

Up to now we have considered waves propagating in an infinite medium so they have never encountered a boundary. The medium for real waves is finite. Strings are only so long and are often tied down at one or both ends. The ripple tank has a wall. When a circular wave in the ripple tank reaches the side of the tank, it seems to bounce off and converge back toward the center of the tank. This observation shows that waves **reflect.** Reflection of sound waves, as we will see in Chapter 2, is an absolutely vital feature in understanding speech production, how musical instruments work, and many other processes in nature. Figure 1-16 ❀ is an "animation" that shows what hap-

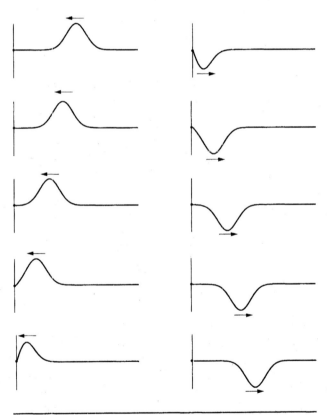

FIGURE 1-16 Reflection from a fixed end. Follow the left column from top to bottom; then return to the top of the right column and follow it downward. A pulse wave moves left on a string whose left end is tied firmly to a wall. When the pulse reaches the fixed end, it stretches the string more than normally, which causes a larger elastic pull than normal, so the pulse will be reflected upside-down back to the right.

pens to an impulsive wave on a string after it hits an end that is tied to a wall. Note that the pulse is reflected upside-down. This feature occurs because the tied-down portion of the string is stretched more than normal when the pulse approaches. The reaction is to cause a larger than normal pullback that bounces the pulse to the upside-down position.

Another kind of arrangement is possible for a boundary. Suppose we let the end move by, for example, tying it to the end of a ring that is free to slide easily up and down along a slippery pole. Then, as we see in Figure 1-17 ❀, the reflected wave comes back right-side-up. Here, the free end gives a smaller than normal elastic pull downward so the rope end simply flops upward. Instead of being held fixed, the pulse now causes twice the normal wave amplitude at the very end, and the pulse returns in the same orientation as it had initially.

Other boundaries besides completely fixed or completely free are possible. When a wave hits an in-

terface between two different media, part of it is transmitted and part of it is reflected. A similar situation occurs when a sound wave attempts to get its signal into the inner ear. Figure 1-18 shows what happens when an impulsive wave traveling on a string encounters a junction after which the string is thicker (more dense) or thinner (less dense) than before. Note that the transmitted pulse is always right-side-up, while the reflected pulse is (a) upside-down if the change is from thick to thin string, and (b) right-side-up if the change is from thick to thin string.

It is easy to see the relation of what happens here to the previous cases of fixed and free ends. The wave

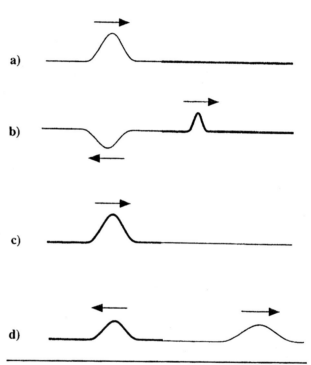

FIGURE 1-18 (a) and (b) An impulsive wave on a light string is traveling to the right to a point that is tied to a thick string. (a) is before the pulse hits; (b) is after. When the pulse hits the boundary between thin and thick strings, some of the pulse is reflected (upside-down) and some is transmitted. Note that the pulse on the thick string moves more slowly than that on the thin string. (c) and (d) An impulsive wave on a thick string is traveling to the right to a point that is tied to a thin string. (c) is before the pulse hits and (d) is after. When the pulse hits the boundary between thin and thick strings, some of the pulse is reflected (right-side-up) and some is transmitted. The pulse on the thin string moves at higher velocity.

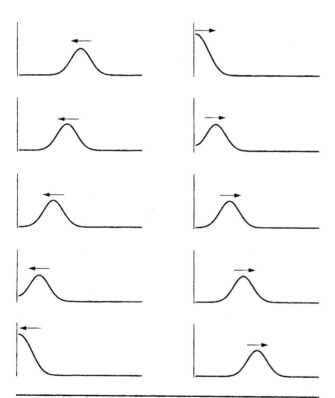

FIGURE 1-17 Reflection from a loose end. Follow the left column from top to bottom; return to the top of the right column and follow that downward. A pulse wave moves left on a string whose left end is free to move. When the pulse reaches the loose end, it simply flops upward, so the pulse is reflected right-side-up back to the right.

traveling on the thin string hitting the thick string is most nearly like the case of an impulsive wave hitting a fixed end (the wall to which a fixed end is tied is essentially infinitely heavy). On the other hand, the second case, where the pulse travels on the thick string, is most like the case of a free end of a string (the case of a completely free end is that of no thin string attached at all). Thus the reflected pulse is right-side-up in this second case. In both cases, the transmitted pulse is right-side-up and is just the original pulse continuing on with diminished amplitude.

❋*ANSWER THIS*

Sometimes you can faintly hear somebody speaking behind a wall in the room next to you because

    a) air molecules penetrate the wall and transmit the sound wave.

    b) sound waves can sneak through tiny openings in the wall.

    c) part of the original sound wave is transmitted through the wall.

    d) the original sound wave breaks apart when it hits the wall, and regenerates itself on the other side of the wall.

    e) none of the above.

1-K. *Interference and Superposition*

The final section of this chapter considers what happens when two waves exist simultaneously in the same region of the medium, as is often the case. For example, consider the ripple tank again. Suppose you dip a finger of one hand into the water in one place and a finger of the other hand at the same time in another place. What happens when the two circular spreading waves meet? The answer, to a very close approximation of the real world, is that the wave forms behave independently of one another. The two circular waves pass through one another. While they are passing through one another, each attempts to disturb the medium in a manner that is completely independent of the other. This property is referred to as the principle of superposition, and it governs the behavior of any waves that overlap or pass through

each other. When two individual traveling waves overlap, the **principle of superposition** states that the shape of the total wave formed is obtained by combining the contributions of the two individual waves. The resulting wave caused by two individual waves could be smaller than, or bigger than, either of the two constituent waves. Once the two waves cease to overlap, they go back to their original shapes. Two waves combining in accord with the principle of superposition are said to **interfere** with one another.

For example, suppose a pulse is traveling to the left and another is traveling to the right. These pulses will pass through each other and, when overlapping, will create a resultant pulse that is the sum of the two individual pulses. Figures 1-19 and 1-20 ❋ show two examples of this type of situation. In Figure 1-19, both

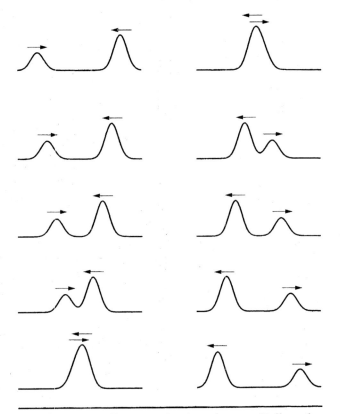

FIGURE 1-19 Constructive interference. Follow the left column from top to bottom; then return to the top of the right column and follow downward. Two positive pulses approach one another. When they meet, both pull up on the string so that, at the time they completely overlap, the maximum height is the sum of the heights of the two pulses. Then they move apart with the same shapes that they had originally.

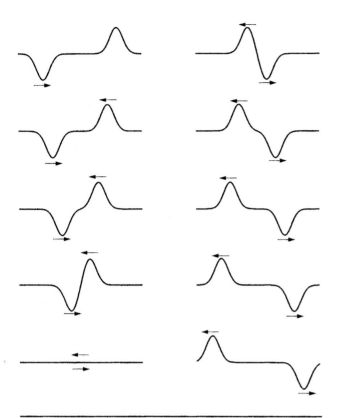

impulsive waves are positive, that is, both displace the string upward. When they pass through each other their effects add, and the total wave is the sum of the two. This adding of waves is called **constructive interference.**

Suppose one of the pulse waves is negative, that is, it pulls the string down. Then the effects of the two waves, when passing through each other, are in opposite directions, and the waves tend to cancel each other. An example is shown in Figure 1-20. This cancellation is know as **destructive interference**.

While we have shown illustrations only for pulse waves, the principle of superposition holds equally well for oscillatory, including sinusoidal, waves. This application will have a very important consequences when we study standing waves in Chapters 2 and 3, wave fronts in Chapter 5, and complex waves in Chapter 6. Without this principle of superposition, spoken or musical sounds would either not exist or would be heard very differently.

FIGURE 1-20 Destructive interference. Follow the left column from top to bottom; then return to the top of the right column and follow downward. A positive and negative pulse approach one another. As they pass through one another, they cancel out temporarily because their sum is zero at that time. Once they have passed one another, they move on without any change in their original shapes.

Exercises

1. A jet airplane takes 2 hours to travel 1800 miles in a straight line. What is the average velocity of the jet?

   a) 1800 miles per hour
   b) 0.0011 miles per hour
   c) 600 miles per hour
   d) 900 miles per hour
   e) none of the above

2. Is the plane in Question 1 supersonic (faster than the speed of sound)? *yes*

3. A grandfather clock ticks once when the pendulum swings from left to right and once again on the swing from right to left. There are two ticks each second. What is the frequency of the pendulum motion in cycles per second (or Hertz, Hz)?

   a) 0.5 Hz
   b) 1 Hz
   c) 2 Hz
   d) 4 Hz
   e) none of the above

4. What is the frequency of the clock in Question 3 in cycles per minute (cpm)?

   a) 20 cpm
   b) 30 cpm
   c) 60 cpm
   d) 120 cpm
   e) none of the above

5. A swimmer standing near the edge of a lake notices a cork bobbing in the water. While watching for one minute, she notices the cork bob (from up to down to back up) 240 times. What is the frequency in Hz of the water wave going by?

   a) 0.5 Hz
   b) 1 Hz
   c) 4 Hz
   d) 120 Hz
   e) 240 Hz

6. Which of the following best describes the water wave in Question 5?

   a) longitudinal
   b) oscillatory
   c) impulsive

7. What is the wave velocity of the water wave in Question 5 in feet per second (ft/s)?

   a) 0.5 ft/s
   b) 1 ft/s
   c) 60 ft/s
   d) 120 ft/s
   e) there is inadequate information to compute the velocity

8. The cork in Question 5 travels 1 foot in moving from its lowest position to its highest position. What is the average velocity of the cork during this motion?

   a) 1 ft/s

   b) 2 ft/s

   c) 3 ft/s

   d) 4 ft/s

   e) none of the above

9. The velocity you found in Question 8 is

   a) the average medium velocity.

   b) the average wave velocity.

   c) neither of these two terms.

10. A student sleeping in class snores 90 times in 3 minutes. What is the frequency of snoring in snores per second (sn/s)?

   a) 0.5 sn/s

   b) 1 sn/s

   c) 2 sn/s

   d) 60 sn/s

   e) none of the above

11. A wave on a rope, at one particular instant in time, looks as shown in Figure 1-21. What is the wavelength of the wave?

   a) 1 ft

   b) 2 ft

   c) 4 ft

   d) 5 ft

   e) 8 ft

12. An explosion might be seen before it is heard because

   a) sound waves have a smaller propagation velocity than light waves.

   b) there is constructive interference.

   c) sound gets fainter the farther you are from where it was created.

   d) friction slows down the sound wave.

   e) a, c, and d are all involved.

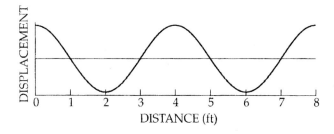

FIGURE 1-21   A wave on a rope at a particular instant of time.

13. Assume that the velocity of sound in air is about 1100 feet per second. A tuning fork that vibrates at 250 Hz gives rise to a sound wave having a wavelength of about

    $1100 = 250 \, \omega$

    a) 0.227 ft.

    b) 4.4 ft.

    c) 250 ft.

    d) 275,000 ft.

14. A pure tone is always

    a) an impulsive wave.

    b) electronically generated.

    c) at very low frequency.

    d) a sinusoidal sound wave.

    e) of small amplitude.

15. Which of the following is false?

    a) The sound waves from two tuning forks of the same frequency will interfere constructively at some points.

    b) Two waves, A and B, have the same wave velocity. If A has a higher frequency than B, A will have a shorter wavelength.

    c) In a transverse wave, the motion of the medium is in the same direction as the wave velocity.

Consider the two graphs in Figure 1-22, denoting the same traveling wave on a string. Problems 16-22 refer to these graphs.

16. The wavelength is

    a) 1 ft.

    b) 2 ft.

    c) 3 ft.

    d) 6 ft.

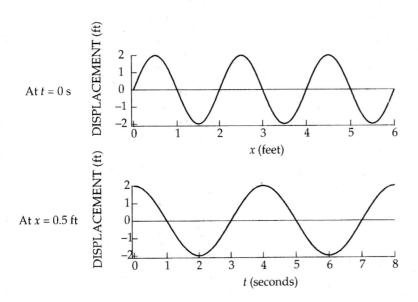

FIGURE 1-22   A wave on a rope versus position is shown at time $t = 0$ in the top part. In the bottom part, the motion at a single position, at $x = 0.5$ ft, is shown as time elapses.

17. The period is

    a) 1 s.
    b) 2 s.
    c) 3 s.
    d) 4 s.

18. The frequency is

    a) 1/8 Hz.
    b) 1/4 Hz.
    c) 1/2 Hz.
    d) 1 Hz.

19. The amplitude is

    a) 1 ft.
    b) 2 ft.
    c) 3 ft.
    d) 6 ft.

20. The wave velocity is

    a) 1/4 ft/s.
    b) 1/2 ft/s.
    c) 1 ft/s.
    d) 2 ft/s.

21. The height of the string at $x = 1$ ft and $t = 0$ s is

    a) –1 ft.
    b) –2 ft.
    c) 0 ft.
    d) 1 ft.
    e) 2 ft.

22. The height of the string at $x = 1$ ft and $t = 4$ s is

    a) –1 ft.
    b) –2 ft.
    c) 0 ft.
    d) 1 ft.
    e) 2 ft.

23. A traveling water wave is described at time $t = 0$ s by the graph of Figure 1-23. The wave is moving to the right and has a frequency of 2 Hz. A bather is in the water at $x = 4$ ft. The swimmer bobs up and down because

    a) of interference effects.
    b) the swimmer has a mass density that differs from the mass density of the water.
    c) the swimmer is surrounded by a medium that moves only vertically.
    d) the wave isn't big enough.
    e) of frictional drag.

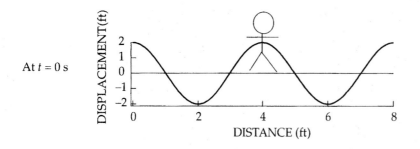

At $t = 0$ s

FIGURE 1-23 A wave in water at a particular instant of time. The swimmer is shown floating at position $x = 4$ ft.

24. At $t = 0.5$ s, the crest that the swimmer in Question 23 was on at $t = 0$ will have moved to

    a) 6 ft.
    b) 8 ft.
    c) 10 ft.
    d) 12 ft.
    e) none of the above.

25. At $t = 1$ s, the swimmer's height above normal surface level will be

    a) –2 ft.
    b) –1 ft.
    c) 0 ft.
    d) 1 ft.
    e) 2 ft.

26. Draw a graph that shows the height of the water at the swimmer's position of Question 23 at $x = 4$ ft as time passes.

27. A can has the air removed by a vacuum pump. The total surface area of the can is 90 square inches. If the pressure of air is 15 pounds per square inch, what is the *total* force on the can's outer surface?

    a) 0.17 pounds
    b) 6 pounds
    c) 15 pounds
    d) 1350 pounds
    e) none of these

28. If I break a piece of chalk having density 0.5 gm/cm³ into two equal pieces, what is the density of each piece?

29. A traveling wave on a string has an amplitude of 1 ft and a frequency of 2 Hz. The wave velocity is 4 ft/s to the right. A point on the string at $x = 2.5$ ft is at a vertical position of 1 ft at time $t = 7$ s. Draw a graph of the displacement of the string as a function of the position along the string (i.e., what would a snapshot of the wave look like at 7 seconds?). Also draw a graph of the displacement of point $x = 0$ as a function of time t in seconds.

2

Standing Waves in Ropes and Strings

In the final sections of Chapter 1, we looked at what happens when a wave meets a boundary and reflection occurs. Reflections at boundaries allow for the possibility of a new kind of wave, called a standing wave because it does not seem to travel in any set direction. Standing waves are at the heart of understanding musical instruments, human speech, and a host of other acoustic phenomena. A good deal of time will be spent considering them and their consequences in the next chapters.

2-A. Formation of Standing Waves

As discussed in Chapter 1, when a traveling wave propagating in a medium encounters an abrupt change in the medium, some reflection and some transmission of the wave occurs. In the case of a wave on a string tied to a wall, all of the wave is reflected (as shown in Figure 1-16). If the abrupt change is due to another string of lighter or heavier mass density, both transmission and reflection occur (see Figure 1-18). Even if the change in the medium is from one having finite mass density to one having zero mass density, such as leaving the end of the string unattached, reflection still occurs; this case is illustrated in Figure 1-17.

Consider a wave-generating machine that causes waves to travel down a string. For a **closed** or **tied** end, the reflected wave is upside-down (Figure 1-16). When the wave encounters an **open** or **free** end, the reflected wave is right-side-up (Figure 1-17). Whether the other end of the string is open or closed, the wave-

generating machine will continuously send pulses down the string, which are then reflected at the other end of the string. The result is a wave traveling to the right (the original wave generated by the machine) and a wave traveling to the left (the reflected wave). Two such traveling waves, one to the right and the other to the left, can generate what we call a standing wave. A **standing wave** is the wave formed by two waves of equal amplitude and frequency traveling in opposite directions. According to the principle of superposition discussed earlier (see Section 1-K), the displacement of the standing wave at a particular point on the string at a particular instant in time is the sum of the two individual displacements of the two traveling waves (see examples of applying the principle of superposition in Figures 1-19 and 1-20). The formation of a standing wave is represented graphically in Figure 2-1.

The sequence of graphs in Figure 2-1 assumes that the wave generator is making the wave at the left (where the vertical axis is), and that the wave is traveling to the right.* The first graph shows where the wave is at a time equal to one period after the wave machine was turned on. Notice that after one period, the machine has generated one complete wavelength. Subsequent graphs show the wave each quarter-period later than the previous graph, except for the last graph, which shows the wave after three periods. Note that after 1.5 periods (corresponding to one and one half wavelengths), the wave hits the wall for the first time. After this time there is a reflected wave. The principle of superposition tells us that the resultant

---

*The amplitudes of all of our diagrams of waves on strings are exaggerated for illustrative purposes. The actual amplitudes that can be achieved in real strings are much smaller.

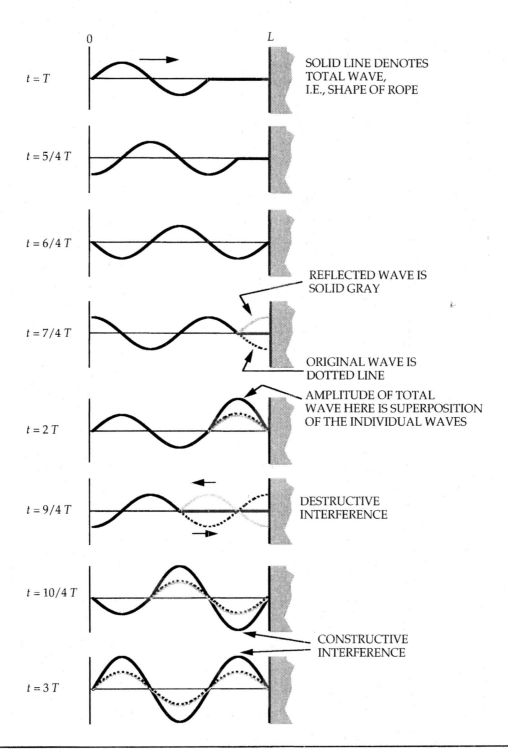

FIGURE 2-1   The formation of a standing wave on a rope. Note that only certain times are shown. A traveling wave moving from left to right hits the wall at time $t = (6/4)T = 1.5T$ in the third frame. After that, there will be a reflected wave traveling to the left (drawn in light gray), and the original wave traveling to the right (drawn as dotted curve), with the total wave, obtained by adding up the reflected wave and the original wave at each point on the string, denoted by the dark black line. Note that constructive interference occurs at points where the total wave is larger than either of the two constituent waves, and destructive interference occurs where the two constituent waves cancel each other.

wave is obtained by adding the two traveling waves at each point along the string. This resultant wave is shown as the solid black line in Figure 2-1.

After the reflected wave reaches the wave generating machine, the shape of the string oscillates, as shown in the Figure 2-2⊛. The wave at the top of each frame in Figure 2-2 is the standing wave that results from adding the original traveling wave to the reflected wave. It is called a standing wave because the peaks and valleys do not travel to the right or left;

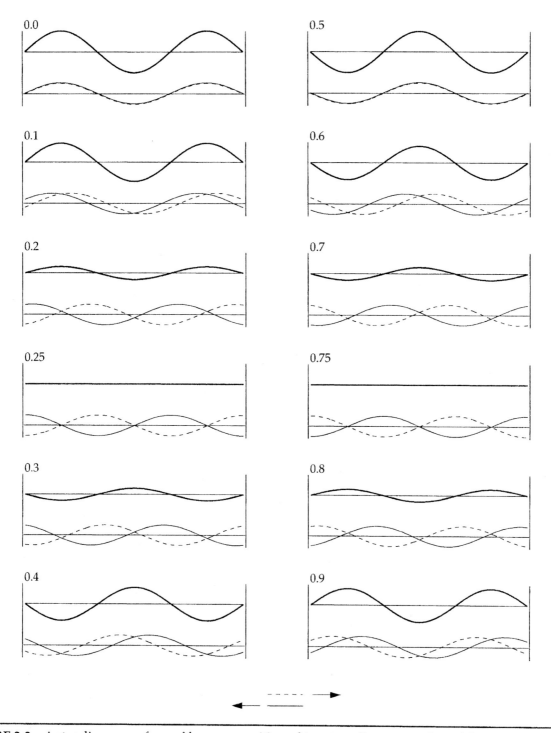

FIGURE 2-2   A standing wave formed by superposition of two traveling waves. One of the waves at the bottom moves to the left, the other to the right. These two waves are added to form the standing wave at the top. This sequence of plots may be seen as an animation at the Web site.

they simply stay at the same positions and oscillate up and down. The bottom part of each frame in Figure 2-2 shows the two traveling waves that contribute to making up the standing wave. One wave at the bottom of each frame is traveling to the right, while the other is traveling to the left. The sum of the two waves at the top of each frame is the standing wave.

Figure 2-3 is a continuation of Figure 2-1 and shows the standing wave at three stop-action time snapshots. Notice that there are points, labeled N in Figure 2-3, and called **nodes,** which are the points where the string does not move at all. The crests and troughs form to the right and left of the nodes, but the node points stay still. Also notice that there are points

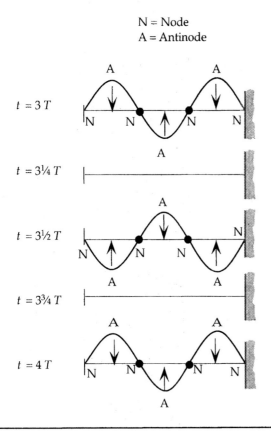

FIGURE 2-3   A standing wave. These five frames show the standing wave of Figure 2-1 for an entire cycle after the standing wave forms, starting at time $t = 3T$ (each frame is one quarter-period later than the previous frame). Note that at each whole or half-period (the first, third, and fifth frames), there is constructive interference and the antinodes of the total wave are at maximum displacement. At each quarter-period (the second and fourth frames), there is destructive interference, and the string is flat, but the string is still in motion even though it is flat.

labeled A in Figure 2-3 called **antinodes,** which are the positions where the displacement of the string is maximum. These are the points where the medium (in this case, the string) undergoes maximum motion as well.

The example we have discussed is for a string that is closed (tied) at both ends. One could construct similar diagrams for a string that is closed at one end and open at the other—in fact, we will do just that below. But first we need to make a brief digression to discuss boundary conditions, which determine the behavior of the string at its ends.

2-B. Boundary Conditions

We have already asserted that, for a given medium, the only wave property that is determined by the medium is the wave velocity; the medium determines the inertial parameter (the linear mass density of the string) and the dynamic parameter (the tension in the string), which in turn determine the wave velocity. Also recall that for a traveling wave, any wavelength or frequency can occur as long as the equation $v = f\lambda$ is satisfied. That is, f and λ can have any value, as long as their product is equal to v.

This situation is not the case for standing waves. When reflections occur at one or both ends of the medium, additional constraints are imposed on the situation. These constraints are called **boundary conditions,** which are the specifications or restrictions on the values that the wave's displacement can have at the **boundaries** of the medium. For example, as in Section 2-A, a string might be tied to a wall at both ends and hence not be free to move at those ends, making the displacement zero at the ends. We will find that, once boundary conditions are imposed, only a special set of wavelengths are allowed on a string. The waves corresponding to these special wavelengths are called **normal modes,** which are simply the set of standing waves that a string (or other wave medium) can support, given the set of boundary conditions imposed. We will now explore a variety of possible boundary conditions to find the normal modes that can be placed on strings and, in the next chapter, those possible in air columns.

2-C. Normal Modes for a String Tied at Both Ends

To start, let's consider a string that is stretched between two rigid walls. Boundary conditions at the

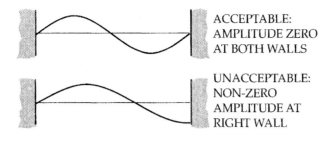

ACCEPTABLE:
AMPLITUDE ZERO
AT BOTH WALLS

UNACCEPTABLE:
NON-ZERO
AMPLITUDE AT
RIGHT WALL

FIGURE 2-4   One acceptable and one unacceptable example of a standing wave on a string with its ends tied.

ends of this string demand that the displacement of any wave shape on the string must be zero at both walls because the ends are tied down and cannot move. Figure 2-4 depicts an example of a situation allowed by the boundary conditions and of a situation that is disallowed by the boundary conditions.

It is important to keep in mind a subtle distinction: Boundary conditions are restrictions placed on the total wave (i.e., the standing wave, which is the sum of the incident and reflected waves). The incident and reflected waves do not have to satisfy boundary conditions separately, as we saw from Figures 2-1 and 2-2.

The effect of boundary conditions is to restrict the possible standing wave shapes to those that have wavelengths that satisfy the following two conditions:

- A **node**, or point of zero displacement, occurs at any closed (tied) end.
- An **antinode**, or point of maximum displacement, occurs at any open (loose) end.

If boundary conditions are imposed at both ends of a string, then one finds that not just any wavelength

is allowed, but rather that the allowed wavelengths form a discrete set. That set of allowed wavelengths determine the **normal modes**, which are the allowed waves on the string. Having a **discrete** set means that only certain wavelengths are allowed; the opposite case, as in the traveling wave on an infinitely long string, is a **continuous** set for which any wavelength is allowed. Figure 2-5 shows the result of applying the first boundary condition above to a string of length L that is tied at both ends to determine its normal modes (only the first four normal modes are shown in Figure 2-5). The pattern shown, in which we choose only waves that have nodes (i.e., zero displacement) at the ends, continues beyond these four in just the same way.

Notice that each subsequent standing wave has one additional antinode and one additional node. The first has only one antinode and two nodes at each end, and its wavelength is $\lambda = 2L$; the reason why the wavelength is twice the length of the string is that half of a wavelength fits into a string of length L (see first diagram in Figure 2-5), and so a full wavelength would fit into a string of length 2L. Moving down to the second standing wave we see that exactly one wavelength fits between the two tied ends, so its wavelength is $\lambda = L$. This wave has two antinodes and three nodes. The next standing wave on the upper right has three antinodes and four nodes; its wavelength is comprised of three consecutive nodes and two consecutive antinodes, so that one whole wavelength fits into a space equal to two-thirds of the length between the walls, and we can write $\lambda = 2L/3$ for the wavelength. As you can see, the allowed wavelengths form a mathematical pattern. If we use the notation, λ_0 (lambda-subzero) to denote the first allowed wavelength, then the entire set of allowed wavelengths can be expressed in terms of λ_0 as follows:

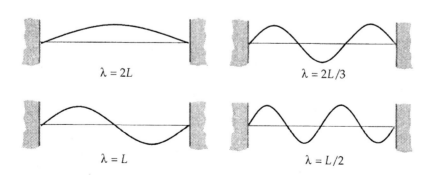

$\lambda = 2L$ $\qquad\qquad$ $\lambda = 2L/3$

$\lambda = L$ $\qquad\qquad$ $\lambda = L/2$

FIGURE 2-5   The first four allowed wavelengths for standing waves on a string tied at both ends. The allowed shapes are determined by demanding that the string remain tied down at both ends. All these allowed waves are examples of what are called the normal modes.

Wavelength for first allowed mode:
$$\lambda_0 = 2L$$

Wavelength for second allowed mode:
$$\lambda = L = \frac{\lambda_0}{2}$$

Wavelength for third allowed mode:
$$\lambda = \frac{2L}{3} = \frac{\lambda_0}{3}$$

Wavelength for fourth allowed mode:
$$\lambda = \frac{L}{2} = \frac{\lambda_0}{4}$$

Wavelength for Nth allowed mode:
$$\lambda = \frac{2L}{N} = \frac{\lambda_0}{N}$$

In the last equation above, N is an integer, which is very convenient for finding the wavelength of any mode. For example, to obtain a value for the wavelength of the seventeenth allowed standing wave (or seventeenth mode), substitute 17 for N: $\lambda = 2L/17 = \lambda_0/17$. Thus, the wavelength of any higher harmonic can be found by dividing the first allowed wavelength, λ_0, by an integer corresponding to the number of the harmonic desired.

❈ ANSWER THIS

Consider the diagram in Figure 2-6 for a standing wave on a string 12 feet long that is tied at both ends. The wave velocity in the string is 16 ft/s. What is the wavelength?

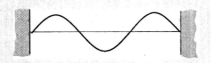

FIGURE 2-6   A standing wave on a string tied at both ends.

For a given medium, the wave velocity and the wavelength determine the frequency of oscillation for the standing wave. Thus, because there is a set of allowed wavelengths, there will also be a set of allowed frequencies, called the **natural frequencies,**

that correspond to the set of allowed wavelengths. Since the wave velocity v, the frequency f, and the wavelength λ, are related by the equation $v = f\lambda$, the set of natural frequencies for sinusoidal waves also form a mathematical pattern. If we denote the first allowed frequency as f_0 (f-subzero), we can write the set of natural frequencies of oscillation for standing waves on a string of length L and wave velocity v as follows:

Frequency for first allowed mode:
$$f_0 = \frac{v}{\lambda_0} = \frac{v}{2L}$$

Frequency for second allowed mode:
$$f = \frac{v}{\lambda} = \frac{v}{\left(\lambda_0/2\right)} = 2\left(\frac{v}{2L}\right) = 2f_0$$

Frequency for third allowed mode:
$$f = \frac{v}{\lambda} = \frac{v}{\left(\lambda_0/3\right)} = 3\left(\frac{v}{2L}\right) = 3f_0$$

Frequency for fourth allowed mode:
$$f = \frac{v}{\lambda} = \frac{v}{\left(\lambda_0/4\right)} = 4\left(\frac{v}{2L}\right) = 4f_0$$

Frequency for Nth allowed mode:
$$f = \frac{v}{\lambda} = \frac{v}{\left(\lambda_0/N\right)} = N\left(\frac{v}{2L}\right) = Nf_0$$

The **first harmonic** is the name given to the first normal mode standing wave in a string, and it has wavelength, $\lambda_0 = 2L$, and frequency, $f_0 = v/2L$. The first harmonic frequency f_0 is also often referred to as the **fundamental frequency**. The second normal mode is called the **second harmonic** or the **first overtone**, and it has a frequency equal to twice the frequency of the first harmonic; the third normal mode is called the **third harmonic** or **second overtone**, and so on. Note that the frequency of any higher harmonic can be found easily in terms of a multiple of the first harmonic by using the last equation above. For example, the fifteenth harmonic has a frequency equal to fifteen times the frequency of the first harmonic.

● ANSWER THIS

Again consider the standing wave in Figure 2-6. The length is still 12 ft and the wave velocity 16 ft/s. Which mode is this? What is the frequency of this mode?

In summary, the first three normal modes for a string of length L that is tied (closed) at both ends, and that has both a tension and a linear mass density such that the wave velocity on the string is v, are shown in Figure 2-7.

In order to change the set of natural frequencies of oscillation of a string tied at both ends one must either change the wave velocity (by changing the tension or the linear mass density of the string) or change the length of the string, L. The allowed wavelengths for a given set of boundary conditions, however, can be changed only by changing L, the length of the string.

The most obvious application of the principles of vibrating strings is the variety of stringed musical instruments, such as violins, cellos, or guitars. In addition to strings, all of these instruments have an acoustical **resonant cavity**, a kind of wooden box that serves to amplify selected frequencies. The properties of this acoustic, or resonant cavity, give an instrument its particular tonal quality. In fact, an auditorium is also a type of resonant cavity, and care must be taken in the design and architecture of auditoriums, otherwise poor acoustics will result. We will return to the topic of resonance in the next chapter.

● ANSWER THIS

For a standing wave on a given string

  a) you can have any λ and any f so long as the relationship $v = f\lambda$ holds.

  b) only certain wavelengths and frequencies are allowed.

  c) the wave velocity is totally determined by the medium.

  d) the wave velocity depends on the dynamic and inertial parameters.

  e) a and c only.

  f) b, c, and d only.

  g) a, c, and d only.

  h) none of the above.

Example: Consider the standing wave in Figure 2-6 again, with length 12 ft and wave velocity 16 ft/s. Exactly how may seconds after the snapshot of Figure 2-6 will the string look like that in Figure 2-8?

Solution: Examine the motion of the string as shown in detail in Figure 2-3. The string moves from its starting point to flat, then to having

(continues)

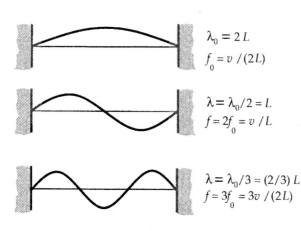

$\lambda_0 = 2L$
$f_0 = v/(2L)$

FUNDAMENTAL FREQUENCY
OR
FIRST HARMONIC

$\lambda = \lambda_0/2 = L$
$f = 2f_0 = v/L$

FIRST OVERTONE
OR
SECOND HARMONIC

$\lambda = \lambda_0/3 = (2/3)L$
$f = 3f_0 = 3v/(2L)$

SECOND OVERTONE
OR
THIRD HARMONIC

FIGURE 2-7 The first three normal modes, wavelengths, and frequencies for a string tied at both ends.

antinodes, then to flat again, and finally, after one period, it returns to its starting point. Thus, to become flat as in Figure 2-8 takes one quarter-period, $T/4$. To find the period, we find the frequency, given by $f = v/\lambda = 16/8 = 2\,\text{Hz}$. The period is $T = \dfrac{1}{f} = \dfrac{1}{2}\,\text{s}$. Thus the time we need is $\dfrac{T}{4} = \dfrac{1}{8}\,\text{s}$.

In fact, the string will again be flat after three-quarters of a period, at $t = (3/8)\,\text{s}$, and so on.

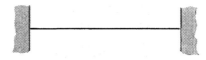

FIGURE 2-8   The string in Figure 2-6, after a time to be determined.

2-D. *Normal Modes for a String Tied at One End and Free at the Other*

Let's next consider the normal modes for a string that is tied (closed) at one end and loose (open) at the other. The boundary conditions depicted in Figure 2-9 must be satisfied. It is difficult to realize the situation shown. It is necessary to get a string to vibrate with a loose end and to still maintain tension on the string under that condition. One possibility is to attach the loose end to a ring that can freely slide up and down along a slippery vertical pole. However difficult it may be to establish this boundary condition, the example we are about to present is important because there are mechanical, acoustical, and electrical analogs of it, including the human vocal tract, and the model is applicable in the real world, as we will see in the next chapter.

Figure 2-10 shows the first three allowed wavelengths on a string of length L that is tied at one end

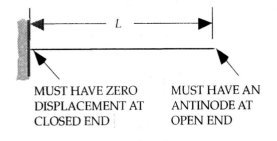

MUST HAVE ZERO   MUST HAVE AN
DISPLACEMENT AT   ANTINODE AT
CLOSED END   OPEN END

FIGURE 2-9   Boundary conditions for a string tied at one end and loose at the other.

and loose at the other. Note that the loose end always has an antinode.

Example: Demonstrate that the wavelength of the fifth harmonic in Figure 2-10 is $(4/5)L$.

Solution: One way to proceed is to divide the wave shape shown into five parts, each one being the distance from a node to an antinode. To make a complete wavelength takes only four such parts, so that the wavelength is four of the five parts of the length, or $\lambda = (4/5)L$.

As before, the allowed wavelengths and frequencies form a mathematical pattern. The set of allowed wavelengths can be summarized as follows:

Wavelength for first allowed mode:
$$\lambda_0 = 4L$$

Wavelength for second allowed mode:
$$\lambda = \frac{4L}{3} = \frac{\lambda_0}{3}$$

Wavelength for third allowed mode:
$$\lambda = \frac{4L}{5} = \frac{\lambda_0}{5}$$

Wavelength for fourth allowed mode:
$$\lambda = \frac{4L}{7} = \frac{\lambda_0}{7}$$

Wavelength for Nth allowed mode:
$$\lambda = \frac{4L}{2N-1} = \frac{\lambda_0}{2N-1}$$

Note that, as was the case for a string tied at both ends, all allowed wavelengths for a string tied at one end and loose at the other can be expressed in terms of the first allowed wavelength divided by an integer; but unlike the previous case, the even integers are skipped (i.e., dividing by an even integer would give rise to an unallowed wavelength since it would not satisfy the boundary conditions). The last equation above can be used to find the wavelength of any allowed mode; for example, to find the wavelength of the fifteenth allowed mode, we divide λ_0 by $(2 \times 15 - 1) = 29$. The allowed frequencies are obtained by divid-

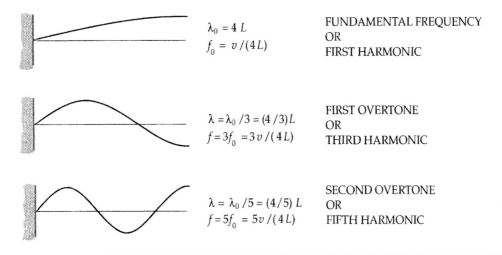

$\lambda_0 = 4L$
$f_0 = v/(4L)$

FUNDAMENTAL FREQUENCY
OR
FIRST HARMONIC

$\lambda = \lambda_0/3 = (4/3)L$
$f = 3f_0 = 3v/(4L)$

FIRST OVERTONE
OR
THIRD HARMONIC

$\lambda = \lambda_0/5 = (4/5)L$
$f = 5f_0 = 5v/(4L)$

SECOND OVERTONE
OR
FIFTH HARMONIC

FIGURE 2-10   The first three normal modes for a string tied at one end and loose at the other end.

ing the wave velocity by the wavelengths and can be expressed as follows:

Frequency for first allowed mode:

$$f_0 = \frac{v}{\lambda_0} = \frac{v}{4L}$$

Frequency for second allowed mode:

$$f = \frac{v}{\lambda} = \frac{v}{\left(\lambda_0/3\right)} = 3\left(\frac{v}{4L}\right) = 3f_0$$

Frequency for third allowed mode:

$$f = \frac{v}{\lambda} = \frac{v}{\left(\lambda_0/5\right)} = 5\left(\frac{v}{4L}\right) = 5f_0$$

Frequency for fourth allowed mode:

$$f = \frac{v}{\lambda} = \frac{v}{\left(\lambda_0/7\right)} = 7\left(\frac{v}{4L}\right) = 7f_0$$

Frequency for Nth allowed mode:

$$f = \frac{v}{\lambda} = \frac{v}{\left(\lambda_0/(2N-1)\right)} = (2N-1)\left(\frac{v}{4L}\right) = (2N-1)f_0$$

As before, the frequency of any higher mode can be found by multiplying the first harmonic, f_0, by an integer, but now we need to skip all even integers.

That is, in a string that is tied at one end and loose at the other, the even harmonics are not allowed; only the odd harmonics are allowed (e.g., the first, third, fifth, etc.). Note that in this type of string, the second allowed mode, or third harmonic, is the first overtone; the third allowed mode, or fifth harmonic, is the second overtone; the fifteenth allowed mode would be the twenty-ninth harmonic and the fourteenth overtone, and so on. The even overtones are not skipped since overtones count all allowed waves after the first.

2-E. Normal Modes for a String Loose at Both Ends

The case for a string open (loose) at both ends is now examined (this case is even more difficult to establish on real strings). Again, we will be more interested in the important analogs to be considered in the next chapter (e.g., an organ pipe is open at both ends).

Figure 2-11 shows the first four allowed wavelengths on a string of length L that is open at both ends that satisfy the boundary conditions that there be an antinode at each end. Notice that, even though the boundary conditions are different and the actual wave shapes look different, the same mathematical pattern for wavelengths emerges here as for a string tied at both ends, $\lambda = 2L, L, 2L/3 \ldots$. Hence, there are only two independent situations for transverse normal modes on a string of length L. They are summarized in Table 2-1.

To summarize, the lowest frequency (f_0) at which a string or rope naturally vibrates is called the first harmonic or fundamental frequency. Any larger allowed frequency is an integer multiple of the first harmonic and is also known as an overtone.

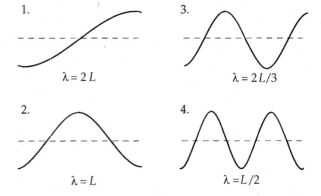

FIGURE 2-11   Normal modes for a string loose at both ends.

TABLE 2-1   Normal Modes for Strings (or Ropes)

Boundary Conditions	Allowed Wavelengths	Natural Frequencies
Both ends loose (open), or both ends tied (closed)	$2L, L, 2L/3, L/2, 2L/5, \ldots$ Wavelength of the Nth allowed wave: $\lambda = \lambda_0/N$, where $\lambda_0 = 2L$, is the first allowed wavelength. N is any integer greater than 1.	$f_0, 2f_0, 3f_0, 4f_0, \ldots$ Frequency of the Nth allowed wave: $f = Nf_0$, where $f_0 = v/2L$, is the first harmonic. N is any integer greater than 1.
One end tied (closed), and one end loose (open)	$4L, 4L/3, 4L/5, 4L/7, 4L/9, \ldots$ Wavelength of the Nth allowed wave: $\lambda = \lambda_0/(2N-1)$, where $\lambda_0 = 4L$, is the first allowed wavelength, and N is any odd integer greater than 1.	$f_0, 3f_0, 5f_0, 7f_0, 9f_0, \ldots$ Frequency of the Nth allowed wave: $f = (2N-1)f_0$, where $f_0 = v/4L$, is the first harmonic, and N is any odd integer greater than 1.

Exercises

A standing wave of a string tied down at $x = 0$ and $x = 10$ ft is described by the graphs in Figure 2-12.

At $t = 0$ s

At $x = 3$ ft

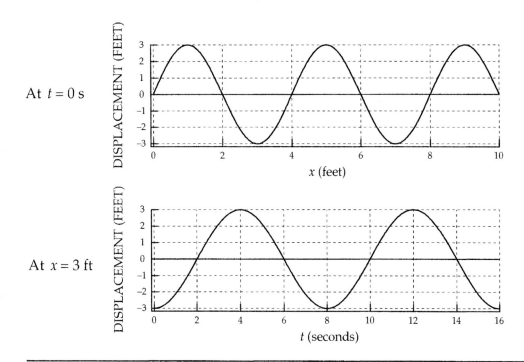

FIGURE 2-12 A standing wave of a string tied down at $x = 0$ and $x = 10$ ft. The top graph shows a snapshot of the string (height versus position) at time $t = 0$. The lower graph (height versus time) shows how the point at $x = 3$ ft behaves with time.

1. What is the wavelength of the standing wave in Figure 2-12?

   a) 3 ft
   b) 4 ft
   c) 5 ft
   d) 10 ft
   e) none of the above

2. What is the amplitude of the standing wave in Figure 2-12?

   a) 3 ft
   b) 4 ft
   c) 5 ft
   d) 10 ft
   e) none of the above

3. What is the period of the standing wave in Figure 2-12?

   a) 4 s
   b) 6 s
   c) 8 s
   d) 10 s
   e) none of the above

4. What is the frequency of the standing wave in Figure 2-12?

    a) 1/16 Hz
    b) 1/8 Hz
    c) 8 Hz
    d) 16 Hz
    e) none of the above

5. What is the wave velocity of the standing wave in Figure 2-12?

    a) 1/2 ft/s
    b) 2 ft/s
    c) 8 ft/s
    d) 16 ft/s
    e) none of the above

6. How many nodes are there in the standing wave in Figure 2-12?

    a) 0
    b) 4
    c) 6
    d) 7
    e) 10

7. How many antinodes are there in the standing wave in Figure 2-12?

    a) 0
    b) 2
    c) 3
    d) 5
    e) 8

8. Which harmonic is the standing wave in Figure 2-12?

    a) none of the below
    b) third harmonic
    c) fourth harmonic
    d) fifth harmonic
    e) sixth harmonic

9. Which overtone is the standing wave in Figure 2-12?

    a) none of the below
    b) third overtone
    c) fourth overtone
    d) fifth overtone
    e) sixth overtone

10. What is the frequency of the second harmonic of the string in Figure 2-12?

    a) 1/40 Hz
    b) 1/20 Hz
    c) 1/2 Hz
    d) 80 Hz
    e) none of the above

11. What wavelength corresponds to the frequency of Question 10?

   a) 3 ft
   b) 4 ft
   c) 5 ft
   d) 10 ft

12. A piece of wire is cut into two pieces, A and B, which are then tightly stretched and mounted between two rigid walls. A and B have the same stretched lengths, but A is stretched more tightly than B. Which of the following quantities will always be larger for waves on A than for waves on B?

   a) amplitude of the wave
   b) frequency of the first harmonic
   c) wave velocity
   d) wavelength of the first harmonic
   e) both b and c

13. A piece of wire is cut into two pieces, A and B, stretched to the same tension, and mounted between two rigid walls. Segment A is longer than segment B. Which of the following quantities will always be larger for waves on A than for waves on B?

   a) amplitude of the wave
   b) frequency of the first harmonic
   c) wave velocity
   d) wavelength of the first harmonic

14. A 4-meter-long string fixed at both ends has a wave velocity of 40 m/s. Which of the following is not an allowed wavelength for a standing waves on the string?

   a) 1/2 m
   b) 2 m
   c) 8/3 m
   d) 10 m

15. A 5-meter-long string fixed at one end only has a wave velocity of 20 m/s. Which of the following is not an allowed frequency for standing waves on this string?

   a) 1 Hz
   b) 2 Hz
   c) 3 Hz
   d) 9 Hz
   e) 101 Hz

3
Standing Waves in Air Columns

The topics discussed in the previous chapter were the allowed transverse standing waves on strings or ropes. Other objects, such as a column of air or a metal rod, also vibrate, but with **longitudinal** standing waves. Earlier it was demonstrated that for a pure-tone (single-frequency) longitudinal sound wave, both the volume mass density (the number of molecules per unit volume) and the pressure vary sinusoidally. Thus far, this has been our only link between the wave concept and sound waves. It turns out that boundary conditions can also be applied to standing sound waves in a column of air, and, as before, this will give rise to **normal modes** (that is, allowed standing waves) in a column of air.

To make the analogy between transverse and longitudinal waves, one must be careful in applying boundary conditions. Remember that in all instances where we have plotted a standing wave on a string, we were plotting the vertical displacement of points on the string. For sound waves, boundary conditions can be applied either to the displacement of air molecules or to the pressure. The pressure and displacement waves are related to each other; however, the boundary conditions given earlier (a node occurs at any closed end, and an antinode occurs at any open end) apply only to sound displacement waves. The boundary conditions for pressure waves are different, as will be discussed below.

3-A. Longitudinal Displacement Waves

When a standing wave on a string is drawn, as in Figure 3-1, it matches the shape of the vibrating string. Another, equally acceptable interpretation is that the wave shape represents how far each point on the string is displaced in the transverse direction from

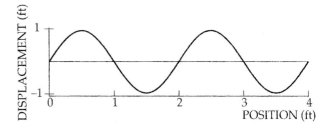

FIGURE 3-1 Plotting a standing wave on a string describes the shape of the string.

its usual (or flat) position. For example, the plot in Figure 3-1 indicates that the point of the string at the horizontal position $x = 0.5$ feet is displaced a distance 1 foot in the vertical (or transverse) direction.

Such **displacement waves** can also represent longitudinal waves, except now the displacement is in the horizontal (as opposed to the transverse) direction. Figure 3-2 displays how a displacement wave for a longitudinal wave should be interpreted. (The numbered balls denote the actual position of

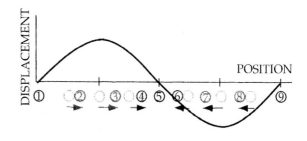

FIGURE 3-2 Interpretation of a longitudinal wave. The height of the plotted line (or wave) is proportional to the distance that each particle moves from its normal position.

particles; "ghost" balls denote their normal positions in the absence of a wave).

The particles labeled 1 and 9 are positioned at end points and do not move at all because they cannot move through the walls. They are "stuck" to the walls. The other particles, except particle 5 which is at a node, are displaced from their normal positions an amount proportional to the size of the displacement wave at that position. That is, particle 2 is displaced from its normal position less than particle 3, so the size of the displacement wave (the height of the wave plot) at particle 3 is bigger than for particle 2. Note that displacement to the right is graphed as positive (see particles 2–4). Correspondingly, displacement to the left is graphed as negative (see particles 6–8).

Figure 3-2 also shows that a rising displacement wave (as occurs in the left-most and right-most sections of the figure) corresponds to a density rarefaction (particles 1–3 and 7–9 are spread farther apart than normal, giving rise to a lower density and lower pressure as well). Similarly, a falling displacement wave (as occurs in the middle of Figure 3-2 for particles 3–7) corresponds to a density compression (the particles are bunched closer together than normal, giving rise to a higher density and higher pressure as well). If the displacement wave is neither rising nor falling, that is, if it is flat (e.g., at the top of the crest and the bottom of the trough in Figure 3-2), adjacent particles are at their normal separations, and hence the pressure is normal there. This can be observed somewhat in Figure 3-2 around the vicinity of particles 3 and 7 (if we had drawn more particles, it would have been more obvious). The boundary conditions to be imposed upon displacement waves for a standing wave in a column of air are now completely analogous to those for transverse waves on a string. Particles near the wall of a tube of air with an end closed cannot be displaced horizontally (i.e., they cannot go through the closed end), just as the tied end of a string cannot move. On the other hand, near an open end of a tube of air, the particles can move horizontally, just as the loose end of a string was free to move. Thus, at an open-ended tube there will be a displacement wave antinode, as occurred at the loose end of the string. This analogy is depicted in Figure 3-3.

Thus, the boundary conditions for a **longitudinal displacement wave** in a column of air are exactly the same as those for transverse waves on a string:

- Closed ends require a node.
- Open ends require an antinode.

We are now in a position to find the normal modes, or permissible wavelengths, that standing

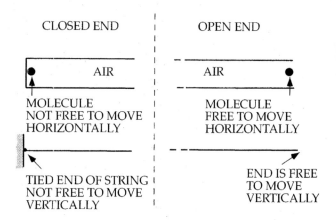

FIGURE 3-3   Illustration of the analogy in boundary conditions between displacement waves in a column of air and transverse waves on strings.

displacement waves can have in an air column. In addition, from the displacement wave, it will be possible to deduce the shape of the pressure wave.

3-B. Normal Modes for an Air Column Closed at Both Ends

This situation, like the case of standing waves on a string loose at both ends, is somewhat unphysical. To get a standing wave on an air column, you usually "drive" it by blowing air into it. However, you can't blow air into a tube that is closed at both ends! But, as was the case for a string loose at both ends, we can proceed and apply the boundary conditions to find the normal modes, since there exist situations analogous to this in the physical world.

Consider the situation in Figure 3-4 of a tube of length L, closed at both ends and filled with air at an average pressure and mass density such that inside the tube the propagation speed of sound is v. The boundary conditions require that there be a point of no displacement at each end. The first four allowed displacement standing waves (i.e., the first four standing waves that satisfy the boundary conditions) are shown in Figure 3-5. Note that these normal

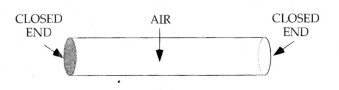

FIGURE 3-4   An air tube closed at both ends.

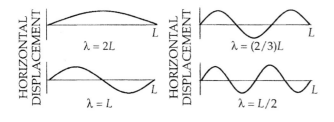

FIGURE 3-5 The first four normal modes for displacement standing waves on an air column closed at both ends.

modes are the same as those of a string with two tied ends.

It is now important to translate what these displacement longitudinal waves would mean in terms of pressure longitudinal waves. Figure 3-6 shows depictions of the first two modes. Since a rising displacement wave corresponds to a density rarefaction (lower density of particles and lower pressure as well), the pressure wave must be below normal pressure when the displacement wave is rising. In fact,

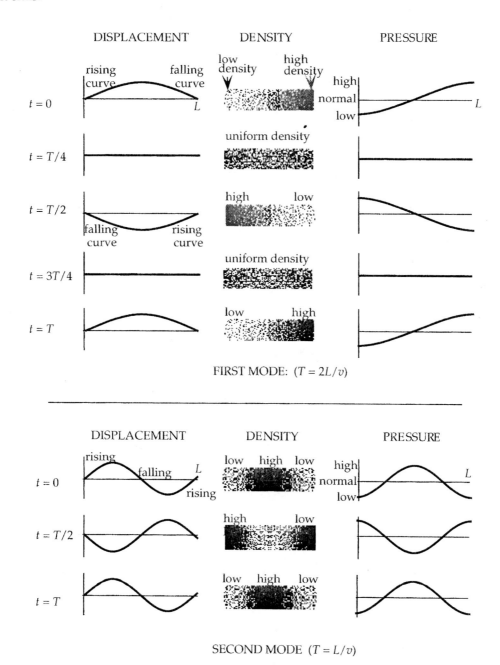

FIGURE 3-6 Correspondence between displacement waves, pressure waves, and density of air for the first two modes of standing waves in an air column closed at both ends.

the steeper the rise in the displacement curve, the lower the pressure. A falling displacement wave corresponds to a density compression (higher density of particles and higher pressure as well); and further, the steeper the fall in the displacement curve, the higher the pressure is above normal. If the displacement curve is flat (neither rising nor falling), the density and the pressure are both normal. One similarity between displacement and pressure waves is that they both oscillate sinusoidally with the same period, frequency, and wavelength. Two important differences between displacement and pressure waves are that

- Displacement nodes correspond to pressure antinodes.
- Displacement antinodes correspond to pressure nodes.

It is often useful to make the connection between displacement and pressure waves by looking at the picture of the molecular "swarm," as in the middle parts of Figure 3-6. Wherever there is a compression, there is obviously a positive pressure antinode. Furthermore, it is clear that molecules must be moving toward that point from either side in order to make the compression, and that at the very center of the compression, there is very little molecular motion. Thus, the displacement there is zero, and to the left side of the compression, the displacement must be positive (i.e., to the right). On the right side of the compression, the displacement, again toward the compression, is negative (i.e., to the left). (Of course, the compression might be at a wall, so one has only one

side to consider.) A rarefaction can be treated similarly. At its middle, there is little molecular displacement and the pressure is at its lowest, corresponding to a negative antinode. Molecules are moving away from that point on both sides, so to the left, the displacement is negative, and to the right it is positive.

3-C. Normal Modes for an Air Column Open at Both Ends

For an air tube of length L that is open at both ends, the boundary conditions for displacement standing waves require antinodes at both ends. The wavelengths for the first four normal modes are shown in Figure 3-8. As was the case for strings, the possible wavelengths for a tube open at both ends are the same as for a tube closed at both ends. Tubes open at both ends are very common in musical instruments (e.g., organ pipes are open at both ends).

Recall that for a given medium, the velocity, frequency, and wavelength are related by the equation $v = f\lambda$. According to this equation, in order to increase the frequency, the wavelength must decrease in order to keep the product constant and equal to the propagation velocity. This type of mathematical is called an inverse relationship, and it is often stated that the frequency is inversely proportional to the wavelength. The implication of this for a musical instrument like the pipe organ is that longer organ pipes have correspondingly longer wavelengths and smaller frequencies than shorter organ pipes. Since the smaller the frequency, the lower the pitch (or conversely, the higher frequency, the higher the pitch), the sounds

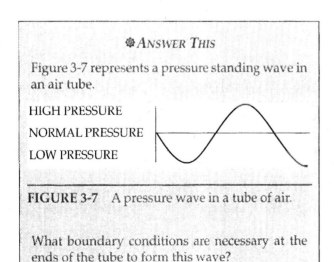

❋ANSWER THIS

Figure 3-7 represents a pressure standing wave in an air tube.

HIGH PRESSURE

NORMAL PRESSURE

LOW PRESSURE

FIGURE 3-7   A pressure wave in a tube of air.

What boundary conditions are necessary at the ends of the tube to form this wave?

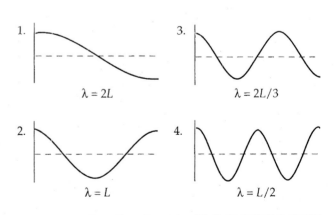

1. $\lambda = 2L$

2. $\lambda = L$

3. $\lambda = 2L/3$

4. $\lambda = L/2$

FIGURE 3-8   The first four normal modes for displacement standing waves on an air column open at both ends.

made by long organ pipes have lower pitches than the sounds made by short organ pipes.

3-D. *Normal Modes for an Air Column Open at One End and Closed at the Other End*

The last case to consider is a tube of length *L* with one open end and one closed end, as shown in Figure 3-9. The boundary conditions on the displacement wave are such that a node must be present at the closed end and an antinode at the open end. The first four normal modes are shown in Figure 3-10.

Remember that these graphs are of the displacement wave, which describes how far air particles are displaced in the horizontal direction from their normal position. The drawings in Figure 3-11 show how the pressure wave is related to the displacement wave for the first two modes for this type of air column. Note that the same set of wavelengths emerge as for a string that was loose at one end and tied at the other end.

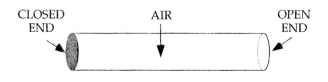

FIGURE 3-9   An air tube closed at one end and open at the other end.

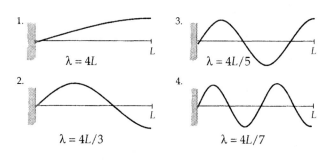

FIGURE 3-10   The first four normal modes for displacement standing waves on an air column open at one end and closed at the other end.

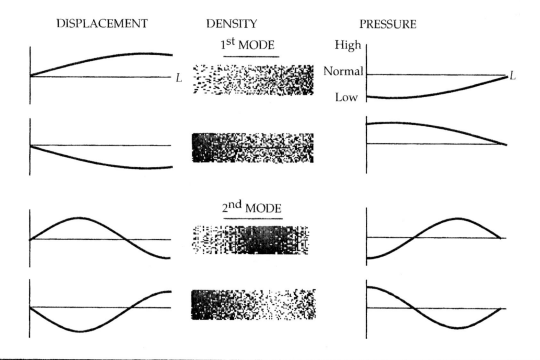

FIGURE 3-11   Correspondence between displacement waves, pressure waves, and density of air for the first two modes of standing waves in an air column closed at one end and open at the other end.

Example: Consider the sound wave of Figure 3-12.

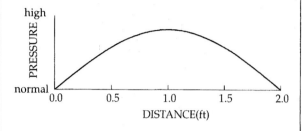

FIGURE 3-12 A pressure sound wave in an air column.

What are the boundary conditions at the ends of the tube? In what direction is the displacement of a particle at position $x = 0.5$ feet? Which harmonic is this? Draw the curve of displacement versus position.

Solution: Because the change in pressure is zero at each end, those ends must both be open (an end open to the whole atmosphere remains at normal pressure). There are corresponding displacement antinodes at each end (because the ends are open, molecules are free to make large movements there). This is a longitudinal wave, so the displacements are *along* the tube either to the right or to the left. There is a compression at the center, so the air molecules are moving toward that position from either end; this means that the displacement at $x = 0.5$ feet is to the right. Displacements at the other half, say at $x = 1.5$, feet are to the left. This mode is the first harmonic; no longer wavelength can satisfy both boundary conditions. A graph of displacement looks like Figure 3-13. Note that the center is a region of falling displacement corresponding to a compression.

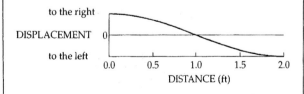

FIGURE 3-13 The displacement curve corresponding to Figure 3-12.

❁ANSWER THIS

An air column with one end open and one end closed is vibrating in its first mode. At a particular instant in time, the air molecules are distributed as in Figure 3-14. Draw the displacement and pressure wave graphs corresponding to this instant in time.

FIGURE 3-14 A picture of the distribution of molecules in a tube with one end open and the other closed.

The advantage of using displacement waves is now apparent. In terms of displacement waves, all media behave the same, and the two boundary conditions cited earlier always hold. The allowed wavelengths are determined only by the boundary conditions and the length of the medium; they do not depend on the medium itself. The wave velocity will, of course, depend on the medium through the inertial and the dynamic parameters. Table 2-1 at the end of the previous chapter also applies to standing waves in a column of air. We repeat Table 2-1 here, calling it Table 3-1, and modify its title to remind us that it holds for strings as well as for air columns.

TABLE 3-1. Normal Modes for Strings and Air Columns

Boundary Conditions	Allowed Wavelengths	Natural Frequencies
Both ends loose (open), or both ends tied (closed)	$2L, L, 2L/3, L/2, 2L/5, \ldots$ Wavelength of the Nth allowed wave: $\lambda = \lambda_0/N$, where $\lambda_0 = 2L$, is the first allowed wavelength. N is any integer greater than 1.	$f_0, 2f_0, 3f_0, 4f_0, \ldots$ Frequency of the Nth allowed wave: $f = Nf_0$, where $f_0 = v/2L$, is the first harmonic. N is any integer greater than 1.
One end tied (closed), and one end loose (open)	$4L, 4L/3, 4L/5, 4L/7, 4L/9, \ldots$ Wavelength of the Nth allowed wave: $\lambda = \lambda_0/(2N-1)$, where $\lambda_0 = 4L$, is the first allowed wavelength, and N is any odd integer greater than 1.	$f_0, 3f_0, 5f_0, 7f_0, 9f_0, \ldots$ Frequency of the Nth allowed wave: $f = (2N-1)f_0$, where $f_0 = v/4L$, is the first harmonic, and N is any odd integer greater than 1.

Exercises

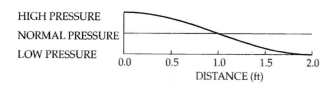

FIGURE 3-15 Pressure versus position in the air tube shown. The tube is 2 feet long.

1. A tube of air has the pressure graph shown in Figure 3-15; the tube must have:
   a) both ends open
   b) both ends closed
   c) left end open, right end closed
   d) left end closed, right end open
   e) I don't know

2. Which standing wave is shown in Figure 3-15?
   a) first harmonic
   b) first overtone
   c) second overtone
   d) third overtone
   e) none of the above

3. What is the wavelength of this standing wave in Figure 3-15?
   a) 1 foot   d) 4 feet
   b) 2 feet   e) 8 feet
   c) 3 feet

4. There is a compression in the wave of Figure 3-15 at
   a) $x = 0$ feet.   d) the position of the node.
   b) $x = 1$ foot.   e) no place in the tube.
   c) $x = 2$ feet.

5. Which of the graphs of molecular displacement versus horizontal distance in Figure 3-16 corresponds to the pressure graph in Figure 3-15?

6. When one blows across the opening of a bottle a tone is heard
   a) only if the bottle contains water so water waves can occur.
   b) because one of the natural frequencies of the air column in the bottle is excited.
   c) because the glass in the bottle carries sound waves.
   d) because air is forced into the bottle and can't get out.

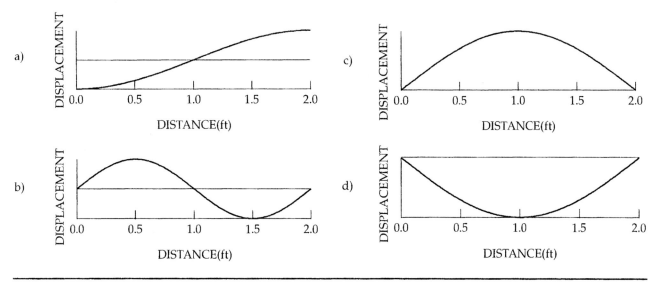

a) DISPLACEMENT — DISTANCE(ft) — 0.0 0.5 1.0 1.5 2.0

c) DISPLACEMENT — DISTANCE(ft) — 0.0 0.5 1.0 1.5 2.0

b) DISPLACEMENT — DISTANCE(ft) — 0.0 0.5 1.0 1.5 2.0

d) DISPLACEMENT — DISTANCE(ft) — 0.0 0.5 1.0 1.5 2.0

FIGURE 3-16   Possible graphs of displacement versus position of a standing sound wave.

7. At a sound wave rarefaction, the

   a) displacement of molecules at either side of the rarefaction is away from the center of the rarefaction.
   b) density is zero.
   c) pressure is above normal.
   d) pressure wave has a node.
   e) displacement wave has an antinode.

8. At the closed end of an air column, there is

   a) a molecular displacement antinode and normal pressure.
   b) zero molecular displacement and a normal pressure.
   c) zero molecular displacement and a pressure antinode.
   d) a molecular displacement antinode and a pressure antinode.
   e) none of these.

9. What are the boundary conditions in a tube of air having the displacement graph of Figure 3-17?

   only odd harmonics

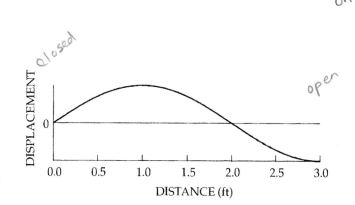

closed

open

DISPLACEMENT — 0 — DISTANCE (ft) — 0.0 0.5 1.0 1.5 2.0 2.5 3.0

FIGURE 3-17   A displacement graph of a standing wave in a tube of air that is 3 feet long.

10. The displacement of a molecule at $x = 1.0$ feet in Figure 3-17 is in what direction?

   (a) to the right
   b) to the left
   c) zero
   d) up
   e) down

11. Which mode is shown in Figure 3-17?

   a) the first mode, also known as the first harmonic
   b) the second mode, also known as the second harmonic
   (c) the second mode, also known as the third harmonic
   d) the third mode, also known as the fifth harmonic
   e) the second mode, also known as the first overtone
   f) both c and e

12. Which of the diagrams in Figure 3-18 best describes the pressure wave graph corresponding to the sound wave of Figure 3-17?

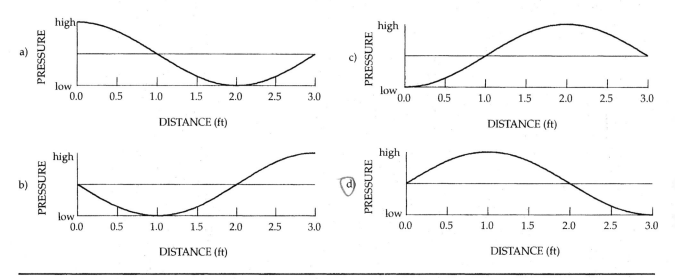

FIGURE 3-18   Pressure wave graphs for Question 12.

13. If the velocity of sound is taken to be about 1100 ft/s, what is the frequency corresponding to the sound wave mode in Figure 3-17?

14. Suppose the displacement graph of Figure 3-17 corresponds to $t = 0$. How much later will the displacement graph be completely flat—that is, will all molecules be at normal position?

4
Resonance

In the previous chapters, we discussed the vibrational states of very simple systems (e.g., strings and air columns). Now that we have classified the possible modes of vibration, we want to discuss how to induce a medium to vibrate in one of its allowed modes. If you want to play a musical instrument whose normal modes make pleasing sounds, it is useful to know how to excite that instrument in the most efficient manner. If you press on the key of a piano, the motion of your finger is passed along to a hammer inside the piano, which in turn hits a string and starts it vibrating. This situation is a general arrangement where sources of motion (e.g., the hammer) pass their energy to some vibrator (e.g., the string). Such an arrangement can be useful in many ways: in changing one type of motion to another (e.g., that of your finger into sound waves via the piano); in taking a random kind of motion and converting it to particular frequencies (e.g., air from a musician's mouth blowing over the opening of a flute, producing the note A); in the amplification of a particular frequency (e.g., placing a tuning fork on a wooden box whose air column amplifies the sound at that same frequency).

In the above paragraph we used the term **energy**, a concept that has deep meaning in physics, although it has not yet been introduced and discussed. It is useful to continue to use the term in the following treatment of resonance even though a detailed development of the idea does not occur until Chapter 10. For now, the concept of energy is used in its most general dictionary definition as the "capacity for action or motion." Thus, when the motion of a finger hitting a piano key leads to the vibration of a piano string and to sound waves emanating from the piano, we speak of energy as having been transferred from finger to string to sound wave. Very often, we can identify energy directly with some motion, so that if a wave has an amplitude, its medium must be in motion, and the

wave has energy. If a sound has a bigger amplitude, it will be louder and contain more energy. The concept of energy can be broader and include forms beyond just motion, however. A small child is said to have a lot of energy when he is moving around in a lively way; however, a sleeping child also has energy in chemical form (food energy) that he can quickly turn into wild motion when awake. In the same way, a drawn bow has such potential energy that can be transferred in an instant to an arrow. Such refinements of the concept of energy will be investigated in more detail in Chapter 10.

We have seen that it is possible to excite a vibrator directly by mechanically disturbing the medium in such a way that it subsequently vibrates. This is what happens when a guitar string is plucked, or an organ pipe is set in one of its vibrational modes by driving air through it, or a piano key is hit by a hammer. Once excited, such vibrators become sources, or generators, of sound waves.

Just as vibrators can behave as generators of sound waves, they can also behave as responders to sound waves, which we will call **resonators**. Under certain circumstances, a vibrator can respond to energy from a sound wave that is traveling by it and start vibrating in one, or several, of its allowed normal modes. Thus, vibrators can be **generators** of sound waves as well as resonators of the energy in a sound wave. Just as a vibrating system (e.g. a string tied at both ends, or an air column open at one end and closed at the other) can vibrate only at certain frequencies called the natural frequencies of oscillation, a vibrator can respond efficiently to a passing sound wave only if the sound wave contains frequencies corresponding to one or more of its natural vibrational modes.

The process by which this energy response (resonance) takes place can be envisioned through a simple mechanical analog. A child on a swing is being pushed by her mother. If the mother pushes the swing at the end of one complete cycle, that is, when the displacement of the swing is maximum, then the amplitude of the swing will become larger with each push. In that case, the frequency of the pushing is the same as the natural frequency of oscillation of the swing. This situation is called **resonance**, which is the increase in amplitude of an oscillator caused by having a **driving frequency** (the frequency of the pusher or energy source) at one of the natural frequencies (normal modes) of the oscillator. In the case of the swing, the oscillator is the child on the swing, and the mother provides the driving frequency by pushing at the right time. Now, if the mother pushes, but not at the natural frequency of oscillation of the swing, then the amplitude of the swing will not increase as much, because occasionally the pusher is actually slowing the swing down by pushing at the wrong time.

The link between the energy source and the energy receiver is not always direct mechanical contact. As we have noted, the linkage might be provided by a sound wave. Consider a traveling sinusoidal sound wave of a particular frequency. Now suppose that this wave is passing by a tuning fork, which is initially not vibrating, and whose natural frequency of vibration matches that of the passing sound wave. As the pressure fluctuations in the sound wave strike the prongs of the fork, the prongs receive a push such that the tuning fork begins to vibrate. Since the frequency of the passing sound wave exactly matches the natural frequency of oscillation of the tuning fork, the successive pushes come at just the right times, and thus the amplitude of oscillation of the tuning fork becomes larger with each push. This is another an example of resonance. Conversely, if the passing sound wave does not have a frequency that matches the natural frequency of oscillation of the tuning fork, the pushes do not occur at the appropriate times, and thus the amplitude increases by only a small amount or not at all. Figure 4-1 depicts the two situations.

There are many naturally occurring instances of resonance. For example, sometimes a singer is depicted as capable of breaking a wine glass just by hitting the right note loudly enough—the frequency of this note matches one of the normal modes of vibration of the wine glass. Thus, the amplitude of vibration of the glass in this mode becomes so large that the glass exceeds its elastic limit and breaks. A famous suspension bridge over the Tacoma Narrows in Washington State collapsed in the late 1930s because the wind excited resonant oscillations of the deck of the bridge.

To repeat the definition in slightly different words, resonance is the sympathetic response of an elastic object and its absorption of energy from a source that has a frequency corresponding to one of the object's natural vibrational modes.

To differentiate the resonating body from the energy source, communication sciences often refer to the frequencies at which the resonator will respond most efficiently as its **natural resonant frequencies.** As before, we continue to refer to the set of frequencies associated with the source as the fundamental frequency and its harmonics. Thus, the fundamental frequency (e.g., the number of pushes on the swing per minute) may or may not match the natural resonant frequency of the responding system (in this case, the swing). The natural resonant frequencies of any responding system will be denoted by F_1, F_2, F_3, and so on. As always, the fundamental frequency of the source is denoted as f_0, and the harmonics as $2f_0$, $3f_0$, and so on. The fundamental physics is not changed here; we have just introduced a notation that clearly distinguishes source from resonator.

Many tuning forks are attached to wooden boxes to amplify their sound. The box usually has one end open and one end closed and is constructed so that the **lowest natural resonant frequency (LNRF, or F_1)** of the air column in the box is precisely tuned to be at the frequency of the tuning fork. When the tuning fork vibrates, its connection to the wood of the box excites the sound wave in the box by resonance; some of the sound leaks out of the open end of the box, and we clearly hear the tone much more loudly than we would from the tuning fork alone. The box has resonated at the tuning fork's fundamental frequency and has acted as an **amplifier** of the sound energy.

Consider such a box (tube), closed at one end and open at the other. As shown in Section 3-D, the frequency of the lowest mode of such a box is $v/4L$, where v is the velocity of sound and L is the tube length. If the box were resonating because of the placement of the tuning fork on it, the LNRF would $F_1 = v/4L$. L would have been chosen so that this frequency matches that of the tuning fork. The higher resonant modes of this box are $F_2 = 3v/4L$, $F_3 = 5v/4L$, and so on. See Table 3-1. Tuning forks of those frequencies could also cause resonance. F_1 is the LNRF, F_2 is then known as the second natural resonant frequency, or simply a higher resonant frequency, and so on.

RESONANCE

SOUND WAVE OF FREQUENCY *f*

INITIALLY NOT VIBRATING
TUNING FORK OF FREQ. *f*

BENDS IN WHEN FIRST
COMPRESSION HITS IT

NEXT COMPRESSION HITS
WHEN PRONGS ARE BENT
OUT

PRONGS BEND IN EVEN
MORE

NEXT COMPRESSION HITS
WHEN PRONGS ARE BENT
OUT

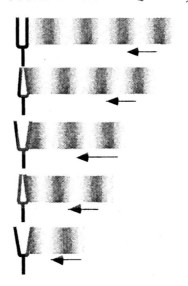

NO RESONANCE
FREQ. OF SOUND WAVE DOES NOT MATCH FREQ. OF TUNING FORK

FIRST COMPRESSION
APPROACHES

PRONGS BEND IN AS FIRST
COMPRESSION HITS

NEXT COMPRESSION HITS
AS PRONGS ARE ABOUT TO
MOVE OUT

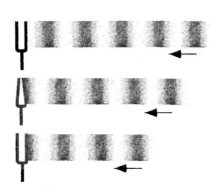

FIGURE 4-1 Cases of resonance and no resonance when a sound wave passes a tuning fork. In the first case, the push provided by the sound wave always comes at the right time. In the second case, sometimes the push slows the tuning fork prongs down because its timing is wrong.

Example: Three pure tones of frequencies 6 Hz, 3 Hz, and 2 Hz are played one at a time near a taut string of length 1 m that is tied at both ends. It is observed that only the 6 Hz tone makes the string vibrate in one of its allowed modes. From this data, what information can we deduce about the string?

Solution: We know that 6 Hz is one of the string's normal modes of vibration, since there is reso-nance at that frequency. If the lowest natural res-onant frequency were 3 Hz, then 6 Hz would be the second resonant frequency; however, the 3 Hz tone would make the string resonate as well, but this is not the case. The 6 Hz frequency can-not be the third resonant frequency either, be-cause then 2 Hz would be the LNRF; nor can it be the sixth resonant frequency with 1 Hz the LNRF.

(continues)

If the latter were the case, then the 2 Hz and 3 Hz tones would be resonant frequencies as well, and would cause vibration. And so on. In this way, we conclude that the string's LNRF must be 6 Hz. Any other alternative would make either 2 Hz or 3 Hz a resonant frequency as well.

Since we know that the LNRF is 6 Hz and that the length of the string is 1 m, we can find the wave velocity on the string by using $F_1 = v/2L$ or $v = 2 L F_1$; $v = 2(1 \text{ m})(6 \text{ Hz}) = 12 \text{ m/s}$. We can also find all the allowed resonant frequencies and corresponding wavelengths: $F_n = n F_1$ and $\lambda_n = 2L/n$, that is, $F_1 = 6 \text{ Hz}$, $F_2 = 12 \text{ Hz}$, $F_3 = 18 \text{ Hz}$, $\dots$; $\lambda_1 = 2$ m, $\lambda_2 = 1$ m, $\lambda_3 = 2/3$ m, $\dots$.

❋ Answer This

Three pure tones of frequencies 12 Hz, 4 Hz, and 3 Hz are played one at a time near a taut string of length 1 m that is tied at both ends. It is observed that only the 12 Hz tone makes the string vibrate in one of its allowed modes. From this information, can you deduce the LNRF of the string? The wave velocity for the string? All the allowed frequencies?

A simple tuning fork can become a generator of sound waves; when it is struck, the prongs undergo sinusoidal oscillations and produce a sound wave. Ultimately, these oscillations die out. Why do they die out? What happened to the energy that the fork had while it was oscillating? Some of the energy of the tuning fork gets dissipated by frictional drag—that is, the prongs of the tuning fork are moving in a sea of air, and as they move back and forth, they drag through the air. **Friction** causes an energy loss because the motion of the tuning fork causes air molecules to increase their random motion. We say that energy has been transferred to the air in the form of **thermal energy**. The situation is analogous to someone treading water in a swimming pool—the arms are moving through the water and thus feel the frictional drag. However, not all of the tuning fork's energy gets dissipated by friction. Some of the energy goes directly into generating the sound wave (i.e., into compressing and rarefying the air). It takes energy to push the air

molecules around and create density fluctuations, and it is the tuning fork that must provide that energy.

Friction also plays an important role in resonance. We might think that if we keep supplying energy to an oscillator, its amplitude would just keep getting bigger and bigger. This does not happen for two reasons:

- We might exceed the elastic limit of the oscillating object (e.g., the wine glass breaks).
- Friction limits the size of the amplitude.

Consider the case of a swinging pendulum in an ideal world without friction. The amplitude, once established by an initial push, would remain the same size indefinitely. A pendulum swinging in air, however, will lose energy by having to push air molecules out of its path. There will also be additional energy losses due to friction in the pivot of the pendulum. Because we live in a world where friction is a reality, we can expect the pendulum swinging in air to have a slowly decreasing amplitude. If we immersed the pendulum in water, we would expect an even faster decrease in the amplitude as time passes, because friction is even greater. The graph below depicts the motion of a swinging pendulum under three conditions: no friction, little friction, and a lot of friction.

The term **damping** is used to describe the frictional loss of energy of a vibrating system. High damping implies a lot of friction, while low damping implies little friction. If a vibrating source having any possible driving frequency, f, is used to excite an elastic object (set it vibrating), we can examine how the amplitude of vibration of the object varies when it is

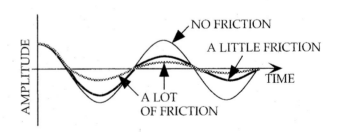

FIGURE 4-2 Displacement versus time for a swinging pendulum. Without friction, the amplitude does not change. With a little friction, the amplitude slowly decreases with time. With a lot of friction, the amplitude drops more quickly. Pendulum energy is lost in heating the surrounding air.

excited by driving frequencies near the object's natural resonant frequency of oscillation, F_n.

Thus, both the amount of friction in the system and the degree to which the source frequency matches the natural resonant frequencies will influence the amplitude of the resulting oscillation. A **resonance curve** is a graph of the amplitude of vibration of the resonator (the degree to which it responds to the energy provided by the source) versus the frequency of the driving energy source. Such a graph will show both the effect of the matching or mismatching of the driving frequency to the resonant frequency and the effect of damping on a system's ability to respond at that frequency. Figure 4-3 is an example of a resonance curve for the swinging pendulum under the three conditions discussed above.

What the resonance curve means is that, if the driving frequency from the source is not tuned properly (that is, if it is considerably less than or greater than the natural frequency F_n), then the corresponding amplitude is very small, as on the left or right ends of the graph. However, if the driving frequency is near F_n (close to the center of the graph), the amplitude can become very large. If there is no damping, one gets the top curve with the unlimited large amplitude. A pendulum immersed in water would not be able to attain a large amplitude even with a constant input of energy because as energy is added, the frictional drag of the pendulum against the water would dissipate the added energy. This situation might correspond to the middle graph. If we now immerse the pendulum in an even thicker liquid, say, light oil, we get even less amplitude for each driving frequency, as in the lowest curve.

It is sometimes useful to view a resonator as a **filter**. A coffee filter allows the good part of the coffee water to pass through and removes the grounds and certain other undesirable elements. In the same way, a resonator emphasizes certain frequencies and removes energy at the mismatched frequencies. It can be said to filter the original vibrating source. More information on filters will be presented in Section 7-E.

Resonance is extremely important to our understanding of many physical phenomena, including, for example, musical instruments and the human voice. The tuning fork on the box is a simple model of a musical instrument. The vibration of the fork at its driving frequency gets the air in the box vibrating at its lowest resonant frequency, and this note becomes amplified. A reed in the mouthpiece of a clarinet vibrates over a range of possible frequencies. When a particular key on the clarinet is pushed, the player is choosing a particular length of the air column in the body of the clarinet. The reed then provides energy at many frequencies simultaneously, but only those frequencies corresponding to the natural modes of vibration of that particular air column get amplified by the air column. The result is a harmonious tone carried by the sound wave escaping from the open end of the tube containing the air column.

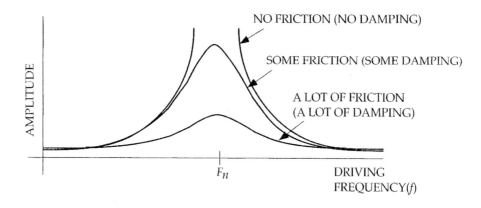

FIGURE 4-3   Resonance curve. Shown is a plot of the amplitude of our resonating oscillator (e.g., a pendulum) as it is pushed by a source that can be run at any driving frequency f. The highest amplitudes occur when f is very close to the resonant frequency F_n of the oscillator. If the driving frequency is off-resonance (f not equal to F_n), the amplitude is smaller. If there were no friction, there would be no limit to how large the amplitude would get at resonance (the oscillator would ultimately break). The more friction there is, the smaller the amplitude is for any given driving frequency.

The human voice works in a similar way, and we will study it in detail in Chapter 8. In very simplified terms, the voice box (the larynx and vocal folds) provide vibrations at a wide range of frequencies; the air column formed between the throat and the lips resonates at particular frequencies. The shape of the vocal tract assumed by the speaker determines which frequencies produced by the vocal folds will be amplified by the resonance of the tract; this shape, in turn, determines which speech sound is produced and heard. Resonance curves like those shown in Figure 4-3 are basic to understanding speech, as we will see in Chapter 8.

Exercises

1. Three pure tones of frequencies 12 Hz, 3 Hz, and 2 Hz are played one at a time near a taut string of length 1 ft that is tied at both ends. It is observed that only the 12 Hz tone makes the string vibrate in one of its allowed modes. From this information, which of the following could we deduce?

   a) the LNRF of the string

   b) all the allowed modes of vibration of the string

   c) the value of the wave velocity for the string

   d) the values of all the allowed wavelengths

2. Three pure tones of frequencies 12 Hz, 7 Hz, and 11 Hz are played one at a time near a taut string of length 1 ft that is tied at both ends. It is observed that only the 12 Hz tone makes the string vibrate in one of its allowed modes. From this information, which of the following could we deduce?

   a) that the LNRF of the string is 12 Hz

   b) that 12 Hz is either the LNRF or one of the other natural resonant frequencies of the string

   c) the value of the wave velocity for the string

   d) the values of all the allowed wavelengths

3. A piece of wire is cut into two pieces, A and B, which are then tightly stretched and mounted between two rigid walls. A and B have the same stretched lengths, but A is stretched more tightly than B. An external driving source that is able to excite the wires is placed nearby. Which of the following could be possible situations? State the circumstances necessary for the item to be true.

   a) A and B have all of the same natural resonant frequencies.

   b) A and B share no natural resonant frequencies.

   c) The LNRF of A matches a higher resonant frequency of B.

   d) The LNRF of B matches a higher resonant frequency of A.

4. A boy has a mass on the bottom end of a spring and, holding the top end of the spring, can shake that end up and down at any frequency he chooses. If he stretches the spring from the bottom and lets go without any shaking, it oscillates at 5 Hz. He shakes his spring end under the following circumstances: in air (a) at 2 Hz, (b) at 5 Hz, (c) at 8 Hz; and then with the mass submerged in a bucket of water at (d) 5Hz. If the amplitude of motion of the boy's hand is always the same, which of these circumstances will result in the largest amplitude of the mass on the end of the spring? Can you tell which situation will have the second largest amplitude?

5. A piece of wire is cut into two pieces, A and B, which are then tightly stretched and mounted between two rigid walls. A and B have the same tension, but A is longer than B. If wire A is plucked and wire B nearby begins to vibrate, it could be because

   a) the fundamental of A is equal to one of the natural resonant frequencies of B.

   b) the LNRF of B is equal to one of the overtones of A.

   c) the normal mode frequencies of A and B are the same.

   d) none of these can be possible.

6. A string of length 2 ft is tied at both ends. When tuning forks of various frequencies are struck near the string, it is found that only the 20 Hz and the 50 Hz forks will start the string vibrating. A knowledgeable friend tells you that the 50 Hz mode on the string is 3 modes higher than the 20 Hz mode. What is the LNRF of the string? What is the wave velocity of any wave on the string?

5

Wave Fronts

In the previous chapter, we showed that waves carry energy, and that under the right conditions this energy can be absorbed by a vibrator through a phenomenon called resonance. In this chapter, we discuss the concept of wave front, which is useful for explaining various wave phenomena, including wave energy, sound intensity, loudness, and constructive as well as destructive interference.

5-A. Wave Fronts

Because we live in a world where friction is a reality, frictional processes ultimately convert all of a wave's energy into thermal energy. (You may wish to review the second paragraph of Chapter 4, where we give a qualitative definition of energy; energy will be treated more rigorously in Chapter 10.) In an idealized world without friction, the situation is much simpler; once created, the total energy in a wave remains constant unless there is some subsequent interaction between the wave and some other source or absorber. The spatial distribution of the energy, however, can change. The distribution of the total energy of a wave throughout the space it occupies at any particular instant in time is determined by the type of wave and the nature of the medium through which it propagates. In the following discussion, we assume that the medium in which the wave travels is uniform—that is, that the average dynamical and inertial properties of the medium do not change as the wave moves through it.

A concept called wave front can help in understanding many wave phenomena, including how wave propagation affects the distribution of wave energy. A **wave front** is that set of points in space for which the wave has maximum amplitude, that is, the crest of the wave. Although the energy carried by a wave is actually distributed throughout the wave, it is

convenient, for purposes of discussion, to consider the energy to be carried by the wave front. The amplitude of the wave front is related to the energy of the wave; if the amplitude of a wave is increased, the energy of the wave at that point increases. A few examples might help clarify this.

5-A-1. One-Dimensional Waves

An example of a type of wave that is confined to move in one dimension is a sinusoidal wave on a string. As the wave in the graph in Figure 5-1 propagates (moves) to the right, the wave fronts (or maxima) move to the right with a speed equal to the wave velocity. In the graph, the wave fronts are marked with little vertical bars.

5-A-2. Two-Dimensional Wave Fronts

Consider a large pool of water with a smooth surface. A two-dimensional wave on this pool can be created by dropping a pebble in the water. The wave fronts in this case are expanding concentric circles, as shown in Figure 5-2. Since the total energy of the wave remains constant (in a perfect world with no friction), and

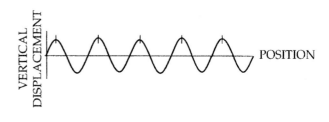

FIGURE 5-1 Wave fronts, denoted by little vertical bars, for a traveling sinusoidal wave on a string. Note that the wave fronts are the crests of the wave.

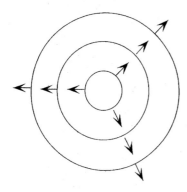

FIGURE 5-2   When a pebble is dropped in a pool of water with a smooth surface, the wave fronts are concentric circles moving outward from where the pebble was dropped.

since the circumference of the circles of the wave created by the pebble are constantly expanding, then the energy per length contained in the wave fronts diminishes as the wave fronts travel outward—that is, the wave's total energy (which is constant) is spread over a larger circumference. Consequently, the amplitude of the wave decreases the farther each wave front gets from the center.

5-A-3. Three-Dimensional Wave Fronts

Three-dimensional waves can be generated in a three-dimensional medium. The only type of three-dimensional wave we will consider are spherical waves. For spherical waves, the wave fronts are spherical shells. As the wave front expands, there is an increasingly larger area over which the energy of the wave spreads. Just as in the two-dimensional case, in order for the total energy to remain constant, the amplitude of the wave fronts will decrease as they get farther from the source. Further, we would expect the rate of decrease to be more pronounced for three-dimensional waves than for two-dimensional waves, because three-dimensional waves spread over a bigger area, while two-dimensional waves spread over a larger circumference. If we try to draw a picture of this on the present two-dimensional page it will pretty much look just like Figure 5-2. You need to think of spheres within spheres within spheres . . . .

A traveling sound wave is a good example of a spherical wave. A tuning fork or a loudspeaker is effectively a point source that generates wave fronts that propagate in spherical shells. The energy is spread over the surface area of the spherical shell. As the shell spreads, the area gets bigger so that the en-

ergy is spread more thinly. It is the **energy per unit area** that determines the **intensity** of the sound, and intensity is related to our perception of loudness. The farther you are from the sound, the thinner the energy spread and the fainter the sound.

Let's consider an analogy. Consider a balloon that has N dots (N is a large number) all over its surface. We are interested in the density of dots on the surface of the balloon, where the density of dots is the number per unit area (e.g., 30 dots per square inch). You may recall from geometry that the surface area of a sphere is $4\pi r^2$. If the radius of the balloon is r, then the density of dots is

$$d = \frac{N}{\text{surface area of balloon}} = \frac{N}{4\pi r^2}$$

If we consider the density when the radius has some different value, say, R, then the corresponding density is D. This density is given by

$$D = \frac{N}{4\pi R^2}$$

The idea is shown in Figure 5-3. The first balloon has a radius of r, and its N dots are spread over a small area. The same balloon is now inflated to a larger radius R and has the same N dots spread over a larger surface area so that the density of dots is less.

If we divide the first density d by the second D, a number of factors (e.g., N, 4, and π) cancel out, making the formula much simpler:

$$\frac{d}{D} = \frac{N / 4\pi r^2}{N / 4\pi R^2} = \frac{R^2}{r^2}$$

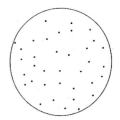

Balloon with N dots   Same balloon with N dots
inflated to radius r now inflated to radius R

FIGURE 5-3   When a balloon with dots painted on its surface is inflated to a larger volume, the dots spread out over a larger surface area, so the density of dots (dots per area) decreases.

Exactly the same argument can be made for the intensity of sound (again, recall that our perception of loudness is directly related to the intensity of the sound wave). The wave energy is spread over increasingly larger spheres as the sound wave spreads out and the amplitude and intensity (related to the energy density) decrease. If the intensity is I_1 when the radius is R_1, and the intensity is I_2 when the radius is R_2, then the two intensities are related by

$$\frac{I_2}{I_1} = \frac{R_1^2}{R_2^2}$$

Note two things:

a) The intensity decreases as the radius increases.

b) The intensity is proportional to 1 divided by the radius squared. It is not a linear proportionality, but a quadratic proportionality.

To see what this means, let us consider Table 5-1. Suppose that you are at a distance of 18 feet from a sound source and that you hear some intensity of, say, $I_1 = 0.04$ Watts/m^2 (the units for intensity are watts per square meter, which is a measure of energy per time per area; this will be discussed more fully in Chapter 10). Now you move twice as far away to 36 feet; the new intensity at 36 feet is one-quarter as much as before. Although the ratio, R_1/R_2 is 1/2, the corresponding I_2/I_1 is, from Table 5-1, 1/4. That is, the new intensity is only one-fourth of 0.04 Watts/m^2, or 0.01 Watts/m^2. If you increase the distance by a factor of 3 the intensity diminishes by a factor of 9, to 0.0044 Watts/m^2, and so on. On the other hand, if you get closer, say, to 6 feet, you are one-third as far away, and the intensity should increase; from Table 5-1 the intensity increases by a factor of 9 to 0.36 Watts/m^2.

Here is another example, which does not use the table. Suppose a point source of sound (say a radio) is adjusted for comfortable listening when you are 3 feet away from it. Another person situated 10 feet away can also comfortably hear the radio. If we represent the intensity of the sound at 3 feet as I_1, then the ratio of the intensity at 10 feet (which we will denote by I_2) to the intensity at 3 feet will be from our formula:

$$\frac{I_2}{I_1} = \frac{3^2}{10^2} = \frac{9}{100} = 0.09$$

Since 0.09 is about one-tenth, this says that the intensity at 10 feet has decreased by about a factor of 10 from the intensity at 3 feet. It turns out that because of the way the sensitivity of the human ear works, this decrease of about a factor of 10 is hardly noticeable to us. In fact, if our hearing were sensitive to intensity decreases of factors of 10 to 100, we would never be able to turn on a stereo in one room and listen to it in a different room. We will investigate how our ear's sensitivity and its determination of loudness depends on intensity in a later chapter.

Example: On July 4, you hear a firecracker go off 50 feet away from you. The intensity you hear is 0.008 Watts/m^2. What intensity would a person who is standing 100 feet away here?

Answer: Since 100 feet is two times farther than 50 feet, the sound intensity at 100 feet should be 1/4 as much as at 50 feet. The intensity at 100 feet is $(1/4) \times (0.008$ Watts/m$^2) = 0.002$ Watts/m^2.

TABLE 5-1   Ratios of Radii and Intensity

R_1/R_2	$(R_1/R_2)^2$	I_2/I_1
1/2	1/4	1/4
1/3	1/9	1/9
1/4	1/16	1/16
2	4	4
3	9	9
4	16	16

❀ *Answer This*

Suppose that later you hear a firecracker go off 60 feet away from you. The intensity you hear is 0.09 Watts/cm^2. What intensity would a person who is standing 20 feet away hear?

a) 0.81 Watts/m^2

b) 0.27 Watts/m^2

c) 0.09 Watts/m^2

d) 0.03 Watts/m^2

e) 0.01 Watts/m^2

5-B. Wave Fronts and Space Interference

Two- and three-dimensional waves can interfere just as one-dimensional waves can. Let us look in some detail now at the interference between two-dimensional waves. The simplest way to see this is to investigate the interference of water waves in a ripple tank. Figure 5-4 shows two sources creating circular two-dimensional waves as they would in a ripple tank; the two sources create the waves by hitting the surface of the water with, say, something like your finger, at a constant frequency. Each set of concentric circles shows the position of the wave fronts (crests of the waves) at a particular point in time. The positions where two wave fronts intersect (where two circles intersect) means that two crests are coming together, thus giving rise to **constructive interference**. At these points of constructive interference, the **total displacement** of the water is the sum of the displacements of the two individual waves. Likewise, **destructive interference** occurs at those places where a crest from one source overlaps a trough from the other source; at these points, there is cancellation of the two waves, and so the total displacement of the water is at a minimum. The lines along which constructive interference occurs can be located by the letters A, B, C, and D in Figure 5-4. They seem to be bright lines if you squint or look at a low angle at the page. The lines along which destructive interference occurs are in between the lettered regions. **Nodal lines** are lines along which destructive interference occurs; the medium is practically still along the nodal lines (a tiny boat sit-

ting on top of a nodal line would hardly bob up and down).

Interference effects are important with sound waves, particularly in rooms or halls used for music or public speaking. In any room, there is always interference between direct sound waves (those that reach you directly from the source) and reflected sound waves from walls or obstacles in the room. Sometimes the reflections can enhance the sound, but they can also detract from sound quality as well. The field of acoustics that studies sound propagation and sound quality in rooms and auditoriums is called architectural acoustics.

5-C. Diffraction of Waves

The final phenomenon related to wave fronts that we will consider is known as diffraction. It arises in everyday experiences. If you talk to someone in the next room with the door open, you do not have to be in line-of-sight with the person to be heard. The sound goes through the open door and bends around the door frame to reach the person. **Diffraction** is the bending of waves around obstacles in their path or the spreading of a wave going through an opening.

Figure 5-5 represents a traveling "wide wave" (technically known as a plane wave) whose wave fronts are depicted in the figure as straight lines. This wave approaches a barrier from the left in a ripple tank and passes through an opening in the barrier.

The wave on the right side can come only from

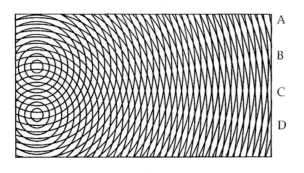

FIGURE 5-4 Interference of circular waves as in a ripple tank. Constructive interference occurs where the circles (crests) overlap; these occur in lines marked at their right ends with the letters A, B, C, and D. Nodal lines, where destructive interference occurs, are in between the lettered lines.

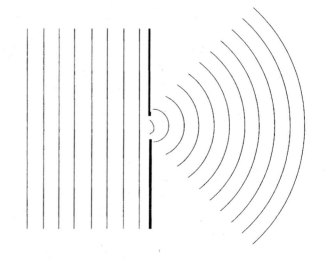

FIGURE 5-5 Waves diffract as they pass through an opening in a ripple tank.

the portion of the wave at the opening. You could imagine what kind of a wave might be generated if one had no plane wave on the left, but instead generated a wave by merely dipping a finger at the appropriate frequency in the water right at the opening. The wave generated would look pretty much like the wave shown on the right of the barrier. It would not be a very narrow plane wave having the width of the opening, but rather would be a circular wave spreading out from the region of the opening. A thorough discussion of the generation of the wave as shown is not as simple as the dipping-finger argument, however; it requires detailed interference considerations that we are unable to consider in this brief survey.

Exercises

1. The intensity of a particular sound at a distance of 10 meters from the source is 0.00009 Watts/m². What is the intensity of the same sound if you are 30 meters away from the source?

   a) 0.00036 Watts/m²

   b) 0.00081 Watts/m²

   c) 0.00003 Watts/m²

   d) 0.00001 Watts/m²

   e) none of the above

2. What is the intensity of the sound in Question 1 if you are 5 meters from the source?

   a) 0.00036 Watts/m²

   b) 0.00018 Watts/m²

   c) 0.000045 Watts/m²

   d) 0.0000225 Watts/m²

   e) none of the above

3. Suppose that Figure 5-4 represents the intersection of wave fronts from two sound sources. If you were to place your ear at the region marked C, you would hear

   a) a sound louder than from either single source.

   b) a sound much less loud than from either single source.

   c) a sound equal in loudness to that from one single source.

   d) a diffracted sound.

4. A certain band's music has an average intensity of 64 microwatts/m² for a listener who is sitting 10 meters away. The listener moves to a distance where the intensity is 4 microwatts/cm². How far away is she now? (In case you are interested, 1 microwatt is 1 millionth Watt; you don't need this information to do this problem, however).

6

Complex Waves

The previous chapters have considered only simple repeating wave forms that are called sinusoidal because they resemble the shape of a mathematical sine function. The corresponding sound wave is a pure tone, which is so simple and relatively uninteresting that it is hardly ever thought of as a musical sound. Most real musical sounds (and speech sounds) involve more complicated oscillatory waves, which appear much richer to our sense of hearing. Any wave that is not sinusoidal is called a **complex wave**. (See Figure 1-3c for an example of an oscillatory wave that is not sinusoidal). If two different musical instruments play the same note, our hearing detects the same pitch, but we are able to distinguish the two notes because they are different complex sound waves.

This chapter will show that a nonsinusoidal repeating wave can be considered to be made up of sinusoidal waves that are related harmonically to one another (e.g., fundamental, second harmonic, etc.). While this analysis is a kind of mathematical trick, it has led to a deep understanding of the nature of complex waves and of the nature of music, speech, and all other sounds. Indeed it has allowed the development of speech recognition devices, as well as speech and music synthesizers. The latter often form complex sounds by adding together several sinusoidal components, the converse of the technique developed in this chapter of decomposing any complex sound into its constituent sinusoidal components.

Our analysis will lead to an understanding of the concept of sound quality, that is, the characteristic of sounds that allows us to detect the difference be-

tween, say, the vowels [ɑ] and [i] (and all other speech sounds) when spoken at the same pitch by the same person. (For an explanation of phonetic notation, see Appendix B.) The fundamental importance of the ideas contained in this chapter and the next to the development of an understanding of speech and hearing cannot be overstressed.

6-A. Phase of a Wave

It is important to understand the term **phase** in order to begin to discuss complex waves. Suppose we have two masses, each hanging on its own spring. The two systems are identical and have the same frequency of motion. If the two masses are pulled down and let go at precisely the same time, they will oscillate in unison. When one is at the top of its motion, the other will be at the top too; when one is at its low point, the other will be at there too, and so on, for each point of their cycles. The two masses are said to be **in phase**. Similarly, two waves are said to be in phase if their cycles are in unison, both reaching a maximum or minimum or other point of their cycles simultaneously. Figure 6-1a shows two waves in phase. Two waves are said to be **out of phase** if their motions are not in unison, as shown in Figure 6-1b. A special case of being out of phase is shown in Figure 6-1c, in which one wave is at a trough when the other is at a crest and vice versa. These two waves are said to have **opposite phases,** or to be 180° out of phase; because these waves have the same period (frequency), they will continue having opposite phases at all later times.

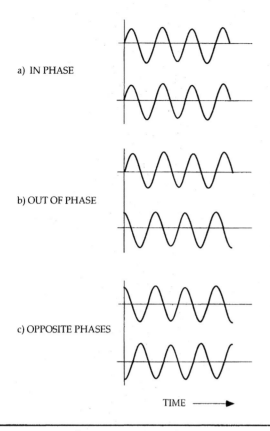

a) IN PHASE

b) OUT OF PHASE

c) OPPOSITE PHASES

TIME ———►

FIGURE 6-1   Illustration of phase relations between two waves. Plotted is displacement versus time *t*. The two waves in (a) are in phase. The waves of (b) are out of phase. The waves of (c) are 180° out of phase; when one is at a crest, the other is at a trough, and vice versa.

6-B. Complex Wave Forms

Suppose we strike two tuning forks of different frequencies at the same instant. The sound wave form that reaches our ear will be a complex wave. Figure 6-3 is a graph of the displacement of a point in the medium as time passes for each tuning fork separately, as well as the resultant displacement that we

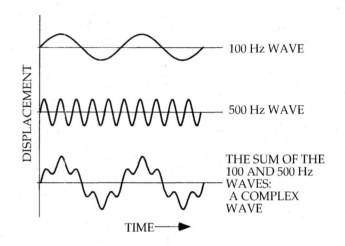

100 Hz WAVE

500 Hz WAVE

THE SUM OF THE 100 AND 500 Hz WAVES: A COMPLEX WAVE

TIME———►

FIGURE 6-3   A complex wave formed by adding two sinusoidal waves together. The top two waves are added point by point to give the total bottom wave by the principle of superposition. The total wave is oscillatory, but not sinusoidal.

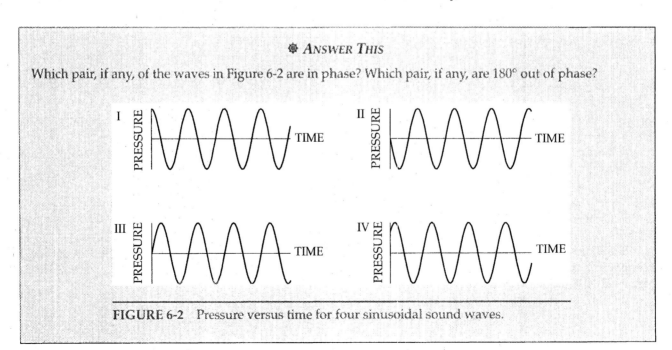

❋ *ANSWER THIS*

Which pair, if any, of the waves in Figure 6-2 are in phase? Which pair, if any, are 180° out of phase?

FIGURE 6-2   Pressure versus time for four sinusoidal sound waves.

get by adding the two individual displacements together at every instant of time using superposition. The lower plot represents the sound wave that reaches the hearer. The total displacement plotted as a function of time is not sinusoidal like the two constituent displacement waves that make it up. However, the total displacement wave is oscillatory because it repeats regularly. In the case corresponding to the graphs, the sound waves from each tuning fork are vibrating so that at some times they are both displacing the air in the same direction and at other times in opposite directions. Thus, at some times constructive interference occurs, and at other times the interference is destructive. The resulting total wave has rather complicated wiggles as a result.

Example: A sinusoidal water wave has a displacement of 0.3 ft at $t = 0$ s and a displacement of 0.1 ft at $t = 3$ s at the side of a boat. It arrives simultaneously with a different sinusoidal water wave having a displacement of 0.1 ft at $t = 0$ s and –0.2 ft at $t = 3$ s at the side of the boat. What is the displacement of the total wave by the side of the boat at each of these times?

Solution: We add the two displacements at each time. The total displacement due to the two waves at $t = 0$ is $(0.3 + 0.1)$ ft = 0.4 ft. At $t = 3$ s, the total displacement is $(0.1 – 0.2)$ ft = –0.1 ft.

6-C. *Complex Traveling Waves*

Let us now look in more detail at the case of how two sinusoidal traveling waves add. Assume that the first wave has a frequency of 200 Hz and the second a frequency of 400 Hz. The 200 Hz wave goes through one complete cycle for every two cycles of the 400 Hz wave. The former has twice the period of the latter. Further, assume that the two waves are both at zero displacement and are rising at time 0. Figure 6-4 shows the two individual displacement waves and the resultant wave that we get by adding the two waves together. (Again, it is important to interpret these graphs appropriately: We are plotting these displacement waves as a function of time—that is, we are plotting the displacement at a given point in the medium as time passes.)

The total wave in Figure 6-4, although not sinusoidal, is oscillatory and has a repeat time equal to

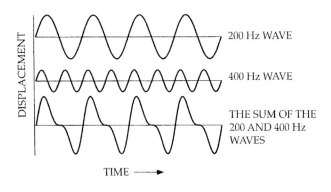

FIGURE 6-4   A 200 Hz wave, a 400 Hz wave, and the complex wave that is the sum of the two. Note the phase of the 400 Hz wave for comparison with that of the next figure.

the period of the 200 Hz wave. That is, **repeat time** is the time it takes the total wave to repeat itself, which in this case is the same as the time it takes the 200 Hz wave (the wave with the larger period) to repeat itself. During that time the 400 Hz wave has repeated itself twice. We used the phrase "repeat time" above rather than "period" when referring to the complex wave because we want to reserve the term "period" for a sinusoidal wave only (i.e., a single-frequency wave). Since period and frequency of a sinusoidal wave are related by the equation, $T = 1/f$, it is not meaningful to talk about the period of a nonsinusoidal complex wave that is made up of two or more frequencies, because in that case two or more periods are actually involved.

Repeat time or its inverse, the **repeat frequency**, which tells us how often the wave repeats its complex pattern, generally determines the **pitch** of the oscillatory sound wave. Like loudness, pitch is a psychoacoustic phenomenon, resulting from the way our brains process the signals received from our hearing mechanisms.

Next, suppose we change the phase of the 400 Hz wave so that the wave is at a maximum at time 0. Figure 6-5 shows the two individual displacement waves and the total displacement wave.

The total wave in Figure 6-5 now looks quite different from the total wave in Figure 6-4. The only difference in the sinusoidal waves of Figure 6-5 compared to those in 6-4 is the slight shift of the phase of the 400 Hz wave. Although these two complex waves look very different, they both still have the same repeat time. But perhaps what is most interesting about the complex waves shown in Figures 6-4

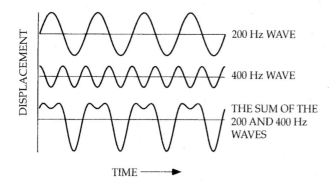

FIGURE 6-5 A 200 Hz wave, a 400 Hz wave, and the complex wave that is the sum of the two. Note that the phase of the 400 Hz wave has been changed from that in Figure 6-4, so that it now has a crest initially.

and 6-5 is that if you were to listen to them as sound waves, they would sound just the same. This is surprising in view of our previous statements that our ears are sensitive to pressure changes; clearly, the ear drum would vibrate differently when the two complex waves of Figures 6-4 and 6-5 came in contact with it. It appears, however, that our hearing cannot distinguish the relative phases of the constituents of a complex wave, a rule known as **Ohm's acoustical law**.

On the other hand, were we to change the amplitude or the frequency of one of the constituent waves, we would certainly be able to detect a difference between the sounds made by the two total waves. (Like most generalizations about hearing, the statement that the ear does not detect phase is not always strictly true. For our purposes, however, Ohm's Law is a good approximation.)

6-D. Complex Standing Waves

Consider the shape of a taut string tied at both ends when it is vibrating in its first two modes simultaneously. Assume that the fundamental frequency is f_0; then the frequency of the second harmonic is $2f_0$. Since the periods are just the reciprocals of the frequencies, the two periods are related as follows:

$$T_{1st\,harmonic} = T_0 = \frac{1}{f_0}, \quad T_{2nd\,harmonic} = \frac{1}{2f_0} = \frac{T_0}{2}$$

Thus, whereas the fundamental will undergo one complete cycle in time T_0, the second harmonic will

❋ ANSWER THIS

Figure 6-6 shows displacement versus time curves for two sinusoidal waves for motion at a particular position on a string.

On the graph plot the complex wave formed by the sum (or superposition) of the two sinusoidal waves.

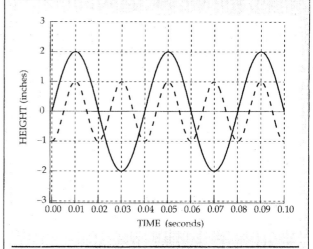

FIGURE 6-6 Two sinusoidal waves to be superimposed on a string.

undergo one complete cycle in half that time (or equivalently, two complete cycles in time T_0).

To explore what the complex standing wave on the string looks like as time passes, let's assume that the amplitude of the fundamental is twice that of the second harmonic. Figure 6-7 shows the two individual constituents (the fundamental and the second harmonic) at different times, and the total wave (the shape of the string) that results from adding the two constituents.

Now suppose that we change the phase of the second harmonic so that it starts at a time $T_0/8$ later. Then the total wave looks different from before. Figure 6-8 shows this new situation.

To summarize, the following factors determine the shape of a complex standing wave on a string as time passes:

- The number and frequencies of the constituent sinusoidal waves making up the complex wave
- The amplitudes of the constituent waves
- The phases of the constituent waves

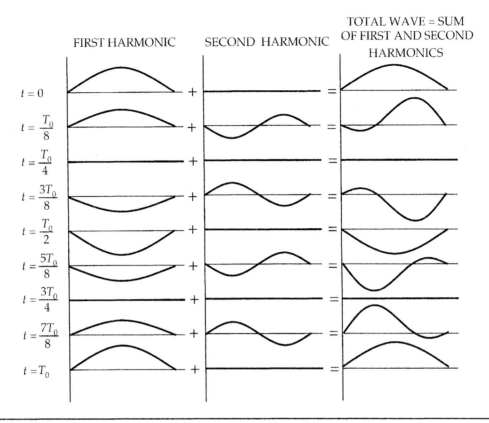

FIRST HARMONIC   SECOND HARMONIC

TOTAL WAVE = SUM
OF FIRST AND SECOND
HARMONICS

FIGURE 6-7   The total wave arising from the sum of the fundamental and the second harmonic standing waves on a string tied at both ends. The vertical axis is displacement; the horizontal is position. Proceeding down the page gives the development at the times listed at the left. T_0 is the period of the first harmonic; the period of the second harmonic is $T_0/2$. On the right is the sum of the two harmonics.

These same three factors affected the shape of a complex traveling wave in the last section. If the string illustrated in Figures 6-7 and 6-8 were a guitar string, we could not tell the difference between the sounds produced in the two cases shown because they result from a differences in phase, which the ear cannot detect.

Example: A standing complex wave on a string of length 2 m is made up of a fundamental of frequency 4 Hz and the fourth harmonic. What is the repeat time of the standing complex wave?

Solution: The period of the fundamental is 1/4 s, which is the time for it to repeat once. The fourth harmonic has frequency 16 Hz (and a period of 1/16 s) and repeats four times during the period of the fundamental. Thus, the repeat time of the complex wave is the period of the fundamental or 0.25 s. The string length is irrelevant to the present example.

Our examples in this and the previous sections have shown what happens when we mix two sinusoidal waves. On a stretched string, one can excite more than just two sinusoidal waves; all the sinusoidal waves of the whole harmonic series are allowed on such a string. So it is no surprise to find that more than just the fundamental mode might be excited if the string is plucked or bowed, as in the case of a violin. Indeed, it is quite consistent to consider that the wave excited by bowing or plucking the string can be considered as a superposition of many harmonics excited simultaneously. Exactly which harmonics are excited, and with what amplitudes, depends on how the string is plucked or bowed. This mixing is done the same way we superposed two waves in the examples described above according to the principle of superposition. Amazingly, we can go much farther and state that any **complex wave,** whatever its origin, **can be considered as made up of a superposition of sinusoidal waves**. We will devote the next chapter to understanding this very important statement.

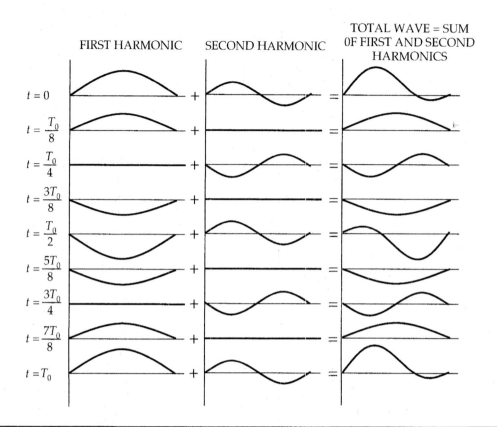

FIGURE 6-8   The total wave arising from the sum of the fundamental and the second harmonic standing waves on a string when the phase of the second harmonic is shifted from the case shown in Figure 6-7.

6-E. Beats

An interesting phenomenon occurs when we form a complex wave from two sinusoidal waves whose amplitudes are the same but whose frequencies differ only slightly. The resulting sound will be heard as a pulsation in loudness of a single tone. These periodic pulsations are called **beats**. As long as the difference in frequency between the two constituent sinusoidal waves is less than 7 Hz, the beats are easily heard. At frequency differences greater than 7 Hz, the beats are not easily discerned, but the sound takes on a sort of rough quality.

The graphs in Figure 6-9 depict the beat phenomenon. Figure 6-9 shows the addition of two constituent sinusoidal waves of exactly the same amplitude, one wave having a frequency of 25 Hz, and the other a frequency of 20 Hz. The total wave shows the regions of constructive and destructive interference. The dashed line shows the **envelope** of the resulting complex wave, and it is this variation of the

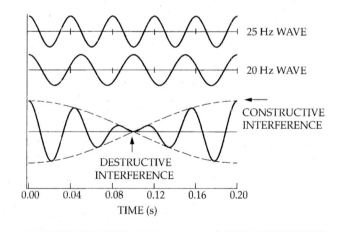

FIGURE 6-9   Beats. When added, two waves of almost the same frequency produce a complex wave whose envelope (shown as the dashed line connecting crests) pulses with a frequency (here 5 Hz) given by the difference between the frequencies of the two component waves.

amplitude with time that we hear as a pulsing sound. The envelope of the figure has a beat frequency of $f = 1/(0.20 \text{ sec}) = 5$ Hz. The fact that 5 Hz is the difference in frequencies between the two constituent sinusoidal waves is no accident. The beat frequency can always be found by subtracting the smaller constituent frequency from the larger constituent frequency; if this difference is less than 7 Hz, beats will be heard.

Note that the waves in the figure are in phase at $t = 0$ since their peaks overlap; there, the amplitude of the total wave is at a maximum. A short time later, because the two waves do not have exactly the same frequency, the constituents slip out of phase and cancel out. They come back into phase again a bit later when their phases match once more. In the example of Figure 6-9, the beat frequency is 5 Hz, with a repeat time of 0.2 s because there is no earlier time at which the two constituent waves will both have completed an integer number of cycles to be back in phase. The 25 Hz wave has oscillated through exactly 5 cycles in 0.2 s, while the 20 Hz wave has oscillated through exactly 4 cycles.

6-F. Sound Quality

We have seen how the addition of two pure sinusoidal waves of different frequencies produces a complex wave. When such a complex wave is heard, the resulting sound is found to be independent of the phase relationship between the two waves. However, if we change either the frequency or the amplitude of either sinusoidal wave, we will perceive a change in sound. One could say that the **quality** of the sound has changed. The terms **timbre, tone quality,** and **tone color** are also used to describe the quality of a sound. Like pitch, quality is a psychoacoustic effect that depends on the reception of the physical sound wave by the hearing mechanism and its further processing by that mechanism and the brain.

Quality is the characteristic of sound that allows two sounds of the same pitch and loudness to be distinguished by the sense of hearing. Very important aspects in determining the quality of a sound are the frequencies and the amplitudes of sinusoidal components in a complex wave.

Two musical instruments do not sound the same even when they play the same note. The wave forms of Figure 6-10, made by a synthesizer, certainly look different from one another. Each tone made, for

example, by a guitar can be considered a mixture of the harmonics allowed on a string, each with a certain amplitude determined by the properties of the instrument and how it is played. The same note played on an clarinet will be made up of exactly the same harmonic series of sinusoidal waves, but with different relative amplitudes. The repeat times of the two notes will be the same because the fundamentals are the same; it is this repeat time that determines the pitch of the notes as detected by our ears. The relative amplitudes of the various harmonics contained in the two tones help determine the sound qualities, which differ for different instruments. We should point out that there are other features, such as attack and decay, that also factor into the sound quality of musical instruments. Attack is the build up of the sound at the beginning of a note, while decay is the fading away of the sound at the end. A recording of a musical instrument played backward will sound like some entirely new instrument, so these are very important elements in music sound quality.

Any particular note has the same fundamental frequency and repeat time whatever the instrument, but the quality depends on the instrument on which it is played and even how it is played. Although each complex wave has its own unique mixture of overtones added to the fundamental frequency, the repeat

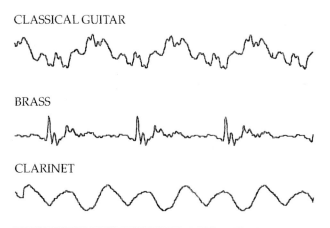

CLASSICAL GUITAR

BRASS

CLARINET

FIGURE 6-10 The complex waves due to some synthesized musical sounds. Pressure is on the vertical axis versus time on the horizontal axis. The entire time scale is about 25 ms. In each case, the synthesizer is playing the same note (at approximately 140 Hz), but the wave forms differ because the waves are made up of different amplitudes of harmonic sinusoidal components.

time (and hence the perceived pitch or note) is the same for all of them since it is based, as we will see, on the period of only the fundamental.

We can apply these ideas to human speech since the human speech mechanism is somewhat similar to a musical instrument. The complex wave produced (in a manner to be discussed in Chapter 8) is a unique mixture of sinusoidal waves of varying frequencies and amplitudes. Our ability to recognize a person's voice and the various speech sounds is based on the quality of the sound produced by the person's voice. The human voice is much more complex than any single musical instrument. By adjusting our vocal tracts, we are able to control the mixtures of frequency components and their amplitudes in the complex wave, making a wave having a unique quality for each speech sound.

Figure 6-11 shows the pressure versus time graphs for the **vowel** sounds "eee" [i], "ah" [ɑ], and "ooh" [u] contained in the words "see," "hot," and "who" and made by the same person. (See Appendix B for a key to the symbols of the International Phonetic Alphabet used in this book.) Not only are the mixtures of overtones different for the various vowels, but they also depend on the speaker. If another person, or the same person at another time, were to record the same vowels, the pressure versus time graphs would be slightly different from those shown in the figure. If we wish to understand the sound quality of speech, we must be much more precise in our analysis of the individual characteristics of sound. This will ultimately lead us to a technique called **Fourier analysis** discussed in the next chapter.

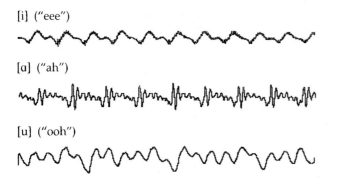

FIGURE 6-11 Waveforms (pressure versus time) for the vowel sounds [i], [ɑ], and [u] in "see," "hot," and "who." All were made by the same female speaker.

> ❈ **ANSWER THIS**
>
> Three complex sound waves are created by adding combinations of frequencies in the harmonic series {$f_0 = 10$ Hz, $2f_0 = 20$ Hz, $3f_0 = 30$ Hz, $4f_0 = 40$ Hz, etc.}. The constituents of the three waves are as follows:
>
> Wave 1 contains first and second harmonics.
>
> Wave 2 contains first, second, and fourth harmonics.
>
> Wave 3 contains first, fifth, and tenth harmonics.
>
> Which of the following is true?
>
> a) The repeat time of all three waves is the same.
>
> b) The repeat time of all three waves is 1/10 s.
>
> c) All three waves may have different repeat times.
>
> d) The repeat time of the three waves depends on the phases of the constituent frequencies, so we can't tell anything about the repeat times.
>
> e) Both a and b.
>
> f) Both c and d.
>
> g) None of the above.

6-G. *Nonrepetitive Sounds*

Up to this point, we have examined complex waves that repeat regularly (i.e., periodic or oscillatory complex waves). Many of the sounds we hear, however, are nonrepetitive. For example, the slam of a car door and the sound made by dropping a book on a table are nonrepetitive sounds. For such impulsive sound waves, it is impossible to identify a pitch with the sound because no one sinusoidal component lasts long enough to impress the ear with its frequency.

Strictly speaking, there are no truly repetitive sound waves at all because all sound waves eventually die out due to friction or because the source stops making them. However, if the wave form is repetitive long enough to convey a sense of pitch, we idealize the wave and consider it periodic in character. As we will see in the next chapter, Fourier analysis will allow us to deal with both repetitive and impulsive waves. The result will be that the only difference between repetitive and nonrepetitive wave forms is the number of constituent frequencies needed to construct the wave.

There is a particular kind of nonrepetitive sound that occurs, at least approximately, quite often. Imagine what you might hear if you played hundreds or thousands of sinusoidal waves, all at the same amplitude, but all with a differing frequencies spread across the audio spectrum. One would expect a chaotic sound with no discernable pitch. Indeed, a composite wave form consisting of an equal amount of every possible frequency is called **white noise**. This type of noise is named in direct analogy to its optical equivalent, white light. White light contains all frequencies of the visible electromagnetic spectrum: violet, indigo, blue, green, yellow, orange, red. A close approximation of white noise is the noise that a television produces when the cable wire is disconnected and you see "snow" on the screen. We have the tendency to think of noise as a waveform of short duration. This is not an accurate way to think of noise. Impulsive waves can indeed be thought of as noise, but not all noise corresponds to a single impulsive wave. A proper definition of noise would be a nonrepetitive sound waveform or, equivalently, a sound

wave for which we can perceive no fundamental frequency. Noise, for example, can be of indefinite duration; Figure 6-12 shows a noise pressure wave resulting from shaking popcorn kernels inside a paper bag. Of course, one might also think of this as many short impulsive waves one after another.

This chapter has shown several examples of complex waves built up by explicitly adding together a few sinusoidal waves. We have also argued that a musical sound could be expected to be made up of several of the possible harmonics produced by the instrument simultaneously. White noise is claimed to be the result of an infinite number of sinusoidal waves sounded together. In the next chapter, we generalize this concept and discuss how any waveform can be broken down into component sinusoidal waves whose amplitude and frequency determine the most important features of the wave.

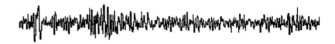

FIGURE 6-12 Waveform of noise (made by shaking raw popcorn in a bag). The wave is nonrepetitive.

Exercises

Questions 1 through 6 are based on Figure 6-6. You should do the problem suggested at the figure.

1. What is the frequency of the wave represented by the solid curve?

   a) 12.5 Hz

   b) 10 Hz

   c) 25 Hz

   d) 50 Hz

   e) none of these

2. What is the amplitude of the wave represented by the solid curve?

   a) 1 in

   b) 2 in

   c) 3 in

   d) 4 in

   e) none of these

3. What is the frequency of the wave represented by the dashed curve?

   a) 12.5 Hz

   b) 10 Hz

   c) 25 Hz

   d) 50 Hz

   e) none of these

4. What is the amplitude of the wave represented by the dashed curve?

   a) 1 in

   b) 2 in

   c) 3 in

   d) 4 in

   e) none of these

5. What is the repeat frequency of the complex wave represented by the sum of the two waves?

   a) 12.5 Hz

   b) 10 Hz

   c) 25 Hz

   d) 50 Hz

   e) none of these

6. What is the repeat time of the complex wave?

   a) 0.04 s

   b) 0.08 s

   c) 0.10 s

   d) 0.12 s

   e) none of these

7. A complex traveling wave can be considered as being composed of

   a) a number of sinusoidal traveling waves differing only in amplitudes and phases.

   b) a number of sinusoidal traveling waves of different frequencies and velocities.

   c) a number of pure tones of different amplitudes but all having the frequency of the complex traveling wave.

   d) a number of sinusoidal traveling waves of different amplitudes and frequencies.

8. When one combines a 230 Hz pure tone with a 233 Hz pure tone, one will hear

   a) white noise

   b) beats

   c) resonance

   d) a pure tone

   e) none of these

9. Two complex wave forms showing pressure versus time, each representing a sound, are shown in Figure 6-13. Which of the following is true?

   a) The two sounds have differing pitches.

   b) The two sounds have the same loudness.

   c) The two sounds have different sound quality.

   d) The two sounds are identical to the ear.

   e) Answers a and c are both correct.

10. A piano tuner uses beats between the note and a tuning fork to tune a piano key. His tuning fork oscillates at 256 Hz, and he hears 3 beats per second. What is the frequency of the piano note?

    a) 3 Hz

    b) 259 Hz

    c) 253 Hz

    d) either 253 or 259 Hz

    e) none of these

11. Changing which one of the following would definitely not affect the repeat time of a complex wave on a string?

    a) the length of the string

    b) the wave velocity

    c) the frequency spectrum

    d) the relative phases of the spectrum components

    e) all of the above affect the repeat time

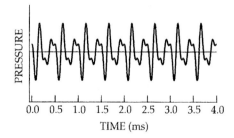

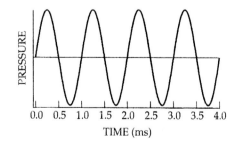

FIGURE 6-13   Pressure versus time plots for sound waves.

12. Applause is best described as which kind of sound wave?

a) pure tone

b) oscillatory complex wave

c) fundamental

d) white noise

e) sinusoidal wave

7
Wave Analysis

In the last chapter, we gave a few examples of the construction of complex waves by the addition of a few sinusoidal waves. A particular wave form is determined if we know the frequencies, amplitudes, and phases of the sinusoidal waves used to construct the complex wave. We intimated that the cases considered were examples of a more general principle, namely that any complex wave could be considered as being built up of constituent sinusoidal waves. We investigate that idea more fully in this chapter. The approach used, called Fourier analysis (after the eighteenth-century French mathematician Jean Baptiste Fourier) will be applied in detail to the study of all sorts of complex waves. The main result of the chapter will be the introduction and use of the idea of the frequency spectrum. In the next chapter, this method will help us understand the speech mechanism.

7-A. Frequency Spectrum

Let us return to the three different vowel sounds in the words s-ee [i], h-o-t, [ɑ], and wh-o [u], whose wave forms were presented in Figure 6-11. An inspection of each graph (had we shown a time axis) would indicate that each of these vowel sounds repeats approximately every 0.005 seconds. This repeat time would suggest that each contains a 200 Hz fundamental frequency. (Review, if necessary, the discussion of repeat time in Section 6-C.). Since the three vowel sounds look different, they must contain other higher frequencies as well. In fact, these vowels all contain harmonics at 200 Hz, 400 Hz, and so on, up to about 1600 Hz, with varying amplitudes for the harmonics for the different vowels. The vowel [i] has no components between 1500 and 2500 Hz (unlike [ɑ] and [u]), but has strong components around 2800 Hz and 4000 Hz. We will study how the human voice

produces the various vowel sounds in Chapter 8 and return to acoustic differences among different vowels in Chapter 9.

Although a change in the relative phase between the components of a complex wave does change the shape of the total pressure wave, as we saw in Figures 6-4 and 6-5, the ear is almost indifferent to such phase changes. The sound that we hear is, to a good approximation, determined only by the amplitudes and the frequencies of the constituent sinusoidal waves. Thus, to characterize any vowel or any other repeating sound, only the frequencies and relative amplitudes of the sinusoidal components making up the vowel sound are needed. For those cases, and for any other complex wave for which phase information is unnecessary, we characterize the wave by just

- The **frequencies** of all the sinusoidal component that make it up.
- The **amplitude** (or amount) of each sinusoidal component present.

This statement is analogous to a recipe for making cookie dough: If we know what ingredients go into the cookie dough (which frequencies are present in the periodic complex wave), and how much of each ingredient to add (the amplitude of each frequency present), we can always make a batch from that recipe of cookie dough (always make the same-sounding complex wave). This observation leads to a convenient way of representing the important characteristics of a complex wave called a **frequency spectrum**, which is usually presented in graphical form. For example, the complex waves drawn in Figures 6-4 and 6-5 consist of two sinusoidal waves of frequencies 200 Hz and 400 Hz, with the amplitude of the 400 Hz wave being one-half the amplitude of the 200 Hz wave. Because we discard phase information, the frequency

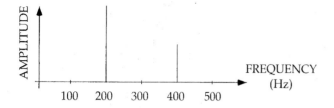

FIGURE 7-1   Frequency spectrum for the waves of Figures 6-4 and 6-5. Each vertical line represents one sinusoidal component in the complex wave. Its height represents the amplitude of the sinusoidal component. The phase of the wave is not shown, so that the graph applies to the complex waves of both Figures 6-4 and 6-5.

spectrum in Figure 7-1 describes both of the complex waves shown in Figures 6-4 and 6-5.

Although the two complex waves in Figures 6-4 and 6-5 look different because of the phase differences in the constituent sinusoidal components, the frequency spectrum looks exactly the same for both. This should not surprise us, because the only piece of information omitted from the frequency spectrum is the phase information, and, since our ears are insensitive to phase differences, the information contained in the frequency spectrum is sufficient to describe uniquely how an ear would perceive a sound.

7-B. Fourier Analysis

To proceed further, we must make use of an extremely important mathematical theorem known as

Fourier's theorem. This theorem is crucial to all fields of science and mathematics involving waves of any kind. Rather than give the precise mathematical statement of Fourier's theorem, we will paraphrase it in terms suited to our needs. We have alluded to the content of this theorem several times already.

Fourier's theorem states that any physically possible complex wave can be represented by a sum of sinusoidal waves having the allowed frequencies. The word "allowed" is used because boundary conditions, if any, will determine precisely what frequencies are allowed. As an example of the application of Fourier's theorem, consider a taut string tied down at both ends. We have already determined the allowable frequencies (normal modes) that the standing waves on this string can have. The first five are reiterated below for convenience.

Now suppose that we deform the string into the triangular shape shown in Figure 7-3 and release it at time 0. It is clear that this complex wave form satisfies the boundary conditions that there is zero displacement at both ends of the string, and that it must continue to satisfy them at later times.

Fourier's theorem can be applied to this situation as follows: We consider this complex wave as made up of many sinusoidal components. Each sinusoidal component would have appropriate amplitudes so that, when all components are added together (using the principle of superposition), the total wave looks exactly like the original complex wave. The subsequent motion of the complex wave can then be determined by studying the motion of the constituent normal modes that make up the complex wave.

The absolute amplitudes of the constituent sinusoidal components (i.e., the exact numerical values of

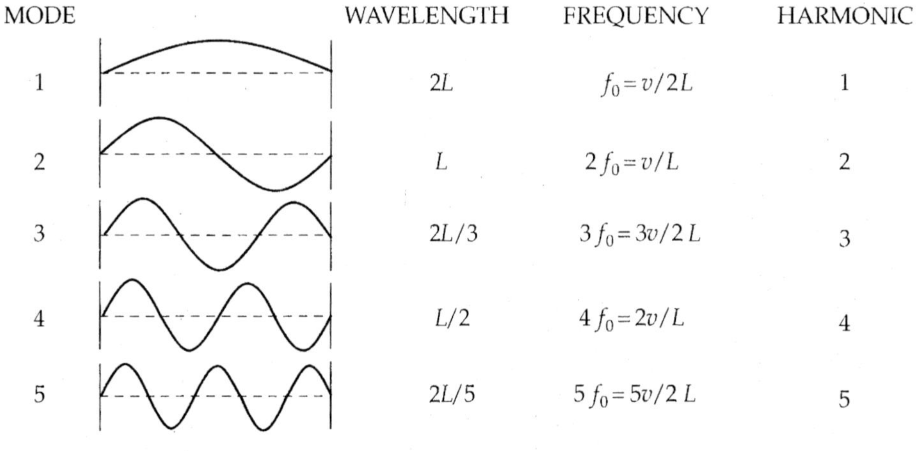

MODE		WAVELENGTH	FREQUENCY	HARMONIC
1		$2L$	$f_0 = v/2L$	1
2		L	$2f_0 = v/L$	2
3		$2L/3$	$3f_0 = 3v/2L$	3
4		$L/2$	$4f_0 = 2v/L$	4
5		$2L/5$	$5f_0 = 5v/2L$	5

FIGURE 7-2   The first five harmonics allowed on a string tied down at both ends.

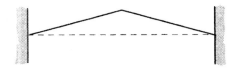

FIGURE 7-3 A possible shape of a stretched string tied at both ends. The string is pulled into this shape and then released at time $t = 0$.

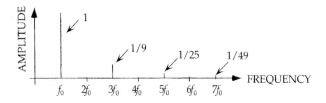

FIGURE 7-5 The frequency spectrum for the triangular wave of Figure 7-4. Note that only the odd harmonics appear, a result that is explained by the fact that the wave shape is symmetrical, that is, the right side is a mirror image of the left side.

the amplitudes) will depend upon the amplitude of the original triangular wave. The diagram of Figure 7-4 shows what happens when we add together the first three constituent modes that are needed to construct the triangular wave according to Fourier's theorem. As you can see, the addition of each sinusoidal component in the series makes the total wave look increasingly like the triangular wave. We have shown only the first three constituent components that are needed to reconstruct the triangular wave. To make the resemblance perfect, we would need an infinite number of modes. However, in practice, including the first few modes will result in a really good facsimile of the complex wave. The frequency spectrum of the triangular complex wave of Figure 7-3 is given in Figure 7-5.

The complex triangular wave of Figure 7-4 is **symmetric**—that is, the part to the right of a vertical line drawn through its midpoint is a mirror image of that to the left of the midline. Another way to visualize this symmetry is to flip one side of the triangular wave using the vertical line through the center as a hinge; the side you are flipping will lie directly on top of the half wave on the other side of the center line. It is no accident that the constituent sinusoidal components needed to reconstruct the complex triangular wave by Fourier's theorem are the odd harmonics, since the odd harmonics are also symmetric about the center point. The even harmonics are antisymmetric about the center point and are not needed to construct a symmetric wave.

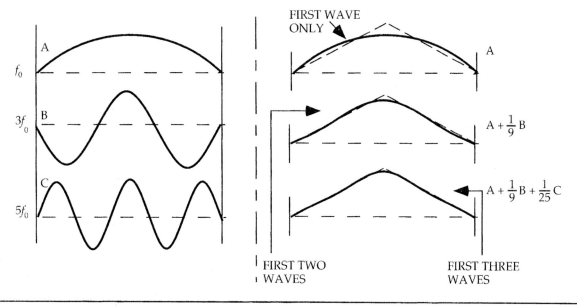

FIGURE 7-4 Fourier's theorem applied to the triangular wave of Figure 7-3. The first three constituent harmonics A, B, and C are shown at the left column. When they are added in the correct amounts, we get a good approximation of the triangular shape. In the right column are shown A alone, A + B/9, and A + B/9 + C/25. Adding more harmonics in the same pattern would reproduce the triangular shape exactly. Determining the precise relative amplitudes is a mathematically complicated problem we do not describe here.

Antisymmetric means that the part to the right is not a mirror image, but is the negative of a mirror image. You need to perform two flips, one from the center line and one from the horizontal line, in order to have the side you flipped lie on top of the half wave on the other side of the center line. Examples of antisymmetric waves are the second and fourth harmonics of the sinusoidal wave shown in Figure 7-2. Symmetry is an important concept in physics, and in Fourier analysis in particular. If the wave you want to construct using Fourier's theorem is symmetric, then only symmetric harmonics will be needed to construct it, which are the odd-numbered harmonics. If the wave you want to construct using Fourier's theorem is antisymmetric, then you need only the antisymmetric harmonics, namely the even ones. A wave of **mixed symmetry** is neither symmetric nor antisymmetric, and both the odd and the even harmonics are needed to construct it. An example of such a wave appears in Figure 7-6.

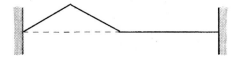

FIGURE 7-6   A wave shape of mixed symmetry. The right half is neither the mirror image of the left half nor its negative.

Figure 7-7 shows the application of Fourier's theorem to the construction of the complex wave of Figure 7-6. The first four modes and their relative amplitudes are shown. Note the odd harmonics denoted by A, C, and D are symmetric, and the those denoted by B and E are antisymmetric. The result is a good approximation of the shape required, but a perfect reproduction would require an infinite number of modes, although with ever-decreasing amplitudes for the higher harmonics.

The frequency spectrum for this complex wave is given in Figure 7-8. Methods of integral calculus are needed to find the amplitudes required to construct this wave shape, so we just quote the results. Note that the fourth harmonic ends up with zero amplitude, so that harmonic is not shown in Figure 7-7.

A periodic or oscillatory wave keeps repeating the same pattern over and over. If you form and release the triangular wave of Figure 7-3, it will, in principle, move down through a rather complicated series of shapes, then move back up to the original shape. (In practice, friction acts on a real string, preventing it from continually repeating the triangular pattern.) The **repeat time** of such a wave is the time it takes to begin repeating the pattern. The **repeat frequency** is the rate (in Hertz) at which the pattern repeats itself. These concepts were previously introduced in Section 6-C.

The repeat time of the triangular complex wave of Figure 7-3 can be found by examining the fre-

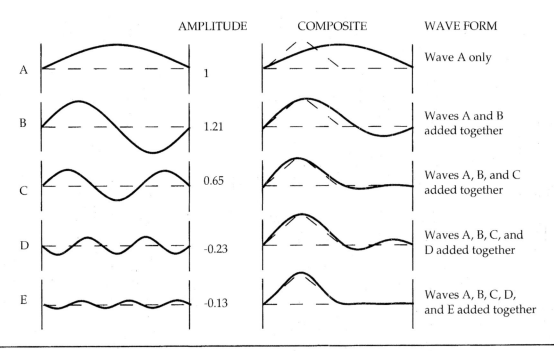

FIGURE 7-7   Building the wave shape of Figure 7-6 by adding harmonics with the amplitudes given in the center column. The fourth harmonic (with five nodes) is missing, that is, it occurs with zero amplitude.

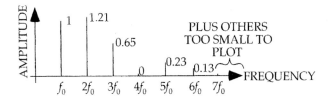

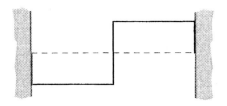

FIGURE 7-8 Frequency spectrum for the wave shape of Figure 7-6. The wave shape is of mixed symmetry, so harmonics of both symmetries are needed with the amplitudes shown.

FIGURE 7-9 A square wave stretched on a string tied at both ends. This wave shape is antisymmetric, and only some of the even harmonics are needed to build it.

quency spectrum. The fundamental, f_0, repeats itself every period, namely every $T_0 = 1/f_0$ seconds. The third harmonic repeats itself every $1/(3f_0) = T_0/3$ seconds, or equivalently, three times every T_0 seconds. Similarly, the fifth harmonic repeats itself once every $T_0/5$ seconds, or five times every T_0 seconds. It follows that for the complex wave to return to its original shape (the triangular shape at time $t = 0$), each component in the Fourier series must return to its original shape. In this case, this happens once every T_0 seconds; that is, the repeat time of this triangular complex wave is equal to the period of the fundamental. Why? Because in time T_0, the fundamental has gone through one complete cycle, the third harmonic has gone through three complete cycles, the fifth harmonic has gone through five complete cycles, and so on, so that all harmonics will have gone through an integer number of cycles, and thus all components of the complex wave have the same shape at time T_0 as they had at $t = 0$. The time T_0 is the shortest time that we must wait until all the harmonics are back to their starting shapes. The repeat frequency and the repeat time of a complex wave are reciprocals of each other, just as the frequency and the period are

reciprocals of each other for sinusoidal waves. Thus, for the triangular wave, the repeat time is T_0, and the repeat frequency is f_0. Repeat frequency is important in sound waves because of its connection to the perception of pitch, as pointed out in the last chapter.

There are cases in which the shortest time one has to wait until the periodic wave repeats itself is shorter than the period of the fundamental. After discussing an example of such a case, we will be able to give general rules for determining the repeat time and repeat frequency. Consider a string that has been deformed, at time 0, into the square wave shown in Figure 7-9. This square complex wave is antisymmetric, because the right half of the wave is the negative of the mirror image of the left half. This feature means that we need only use antisymmetric modes, which are the even harmonics to build the wave. The first frequency needed to construct this complex wave according to Fourier's theorem is $2f_0$, where f_0 is the fundamental frequency of the string (recall the relationship, nth harmonic = nf_0). It turns out (as found by means involving calculus) that we need the second, sixth, tenth, fourteenth, and so on harmonics to build up this complex wave. Figure 7-10 shows how the total

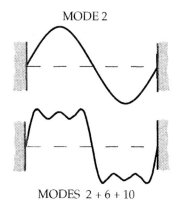

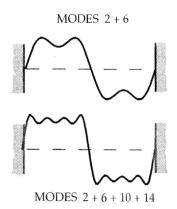

FIGURE 7-10 The construction by Fourier analysis of the square wave of Figure 7-9. Only certain even harmonics are needed to build it. To make it look just like the square wave would require an infinite number of modes with decreasing amplitudes for higher mode numbers.

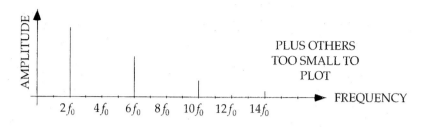

FIGURE 7-11   The frequency spectrum for the square wave of Figure 7-9.

wave would look as we keep adding the necessary harmonics. The frequency spectrum of the square wave appears in Figure 7-11.

For this particular example, we do not need the odd harmonics (or even the alternate even harmonics) to build this wave. Since all of the harmonics needed are integer multiples of the second harmonic, the repeat frequency of the complex square wave will be $2f_0$, and the repeat time of the complex wave will be $T_{\text{repeat}} = 1/(2f_0) = T_0/2$, that is, half the period of the fundamental. In other words, in time $T_{\text{repeat}} = T_0/2$, the second harmonic will go through one complete cycle, the sixth harmonic will go through three complete cycles, the tenth harmonic will go through five complete cycles, and so on, so that, after that time, all components add up to the same shape that the original square wave had at time 0. This is an example of a complex wave whose repeat time is not equal to the period of the fundamental, but is less than the fundamental's period. In this case, the second harmonic acts to the other components rather like a fundamental does; that is, all the other frequencies are integer multiples of it, and $2f_0$ is the largest common factor of the other frequencies. There is no larger number that, when multiplied by various integers, gives all the other frequencies present. In Section 7-C, we review what we have learned about repeat frequencies and repeat times and formulate a simple set of rules for computing these quantities.

The examples we have considered so far all have one thing in common, namely, that the largest amplitude component in the frequency spectrum corresponds to the lowest frequency. This need not be the case. Suppose we have a complex wave consisting of a high-frequency region positioned at the center of the string at time 0, as shown in Figure 7-12. To be more definite, assume that the wiggle in the middle of the complex wave shown is a segment of the thirty-ninth harmonic. Since this complex wave is symmetric, a small amount of the first mode is needed. It

should be clear, however, that the largest amplitude component in the frequency spectrum will be the thirty-ninth harmonic, since the thirty-ninth harmonic looks most like the complex wave we want to reconstruct, and hence more of this component is needed than the others. This complex wave will have a frequency spectrum something like the one in Figure 7-13.

Although the largest amplitude frequency component is $39f_0$, the repeat time of the wave is still the period of the fundamental, T_0, because there is a little bit of the fundamental frequency in the frequency spectrum of this complex wave, and the first time all harmonics can repeat in unison is after the period of the fundamental.

As mentioned, finding exactly what relative amplitudes are needed for the harmonics used to build a complex wave would require considerable mathematical sophistication, including integral calculus. However, even without such detailed information, we have shown how it is possible to discuss many general features of the components of the complex wave. For example, we saw how symmetry can be used to determine the types of harmonics needed (odd, even, or both); we also saw how we can usually determine the repeat time and repeat frequency of various complex waves from general properties.

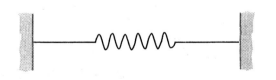

FIGURE 7-12   A complex wave, the middle of which at $t = 0$ is a piece of a high harmonic and zero to either side.

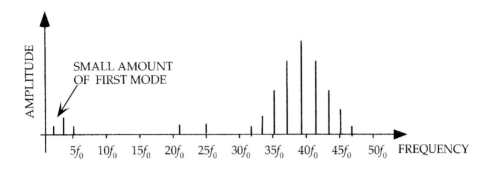

FIGURE 7-13   Approximate frequency spectrum for the wave shape of Figure 7-12.

Example: Figure 7-14 shows a string stretched into a particular shape. Which of the frequency spectra in the figure is most likely to describe this wave shape?

Solution: Because the wave is symmetric, the wave spectrum contains only the symmetric harmonics, which are the odd harmonics, f_0, $3f_0$, $5f_0$, etc. Thus a and b are eliminated as possible answers. Note that the wave shape has two nodes and looks a lot like the third harmonic; we expect that the amplitude of the third harmonic, $3f_0$, will dominate the spectrum as it does in d, which is the correct answer.

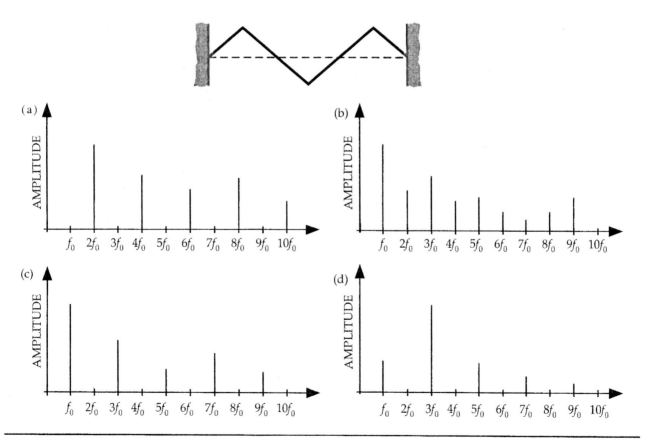

FIGURE 7-14   A wave shape and some possible frequency spectra to describe it. The labels on the horizontal axis (f_0, $2f_0$, etc.) refer to harmonics of the string shown.

7-C. *Behavior of the String with Time*

In the previous section, we described how we can construct a complex wave having a particular shape at time $t = 0$, and we considered several complex wave shapes on a string. Suppose we release the string having one of the shapes given in the examples. Each of the sinusoidal components moves according to its usual motion as a standing wave. The overall shape of the string at any time, then, can be found by allowing each component to change separately with time, then adding up all components using the superposition principle. This motion can be exceedingly complicated and not particularly easy to find without elaborate mathematical methods. We do know, however, that after what may be a complicated motion, the ideal string will return to its starting shape. (In real strings, friction usually damps out the higher-frequency harmonics first, so the shape does not return to exactly the same form each time.) As an example of the oscillation of a string with time for a complex wave shape, we illustrate the motion of the square shape of Figure 7-9. Figure 7-15 shows the shape of the wave every eighth of the repeat time, T, where T, in this case of an antisymmetric wave, is the period of the second harmonic.

❀ ANSWER THIS

Explain why the wave shape is flat (zero displacement) at $t = 3T/4$ and $T/4$ in Figure 7-15. Why is it the negative of its original shape at $t = T/2$?

The shape initially breaks up into two little square pulses that move apart, collide with the walls, reflect (upside down), rejoin at the center, and so on. An animation of this is shown on the Web site. ❀

7-D. *Rules for Repeat Frequencies of Complex Waves*

Among the most important aspects of a complex wave are its repeat time and its reciprocal, the repeat frequency. The latter determines the pitch of a complex sound wave. From Fourier's theorem, we know that any complex standing wave on a string can be written as a sum of components, where each component consists of a normal mode having the appropriate amplitude. Since the possible frequencies on a string tied at both ends form a **harmonic series** $\{f_0, 2f_0, 3f_0, 4f_0, \ldots\}$ we know that the repeat time of any complex wave on the string cannot be longer than the period of the fundamental, T_0. The reason is that T_0 is the longest period of all the frequencies in the harmonic series. The period of any higher harmonic (say the nth one) can be written as T_0/n, which means that the nth harmonic goes through n complete cycles in the time that the fundamental goes through only one complete cycle, so we would have to wait at least that time, T_0, for the complex wave to repeat itself. However, we saw that the repeat time can be shorter than T_0, depending on the frequencies needed to construct the complete wave. If all the needed frequencies are multiples of the lowest frequency in the frequency spectrum, the repeat time of the complex wave is equal to the period of the lowest mode appearing in the Fourier series. The examples studied so far are summarized in Figure 7-16.

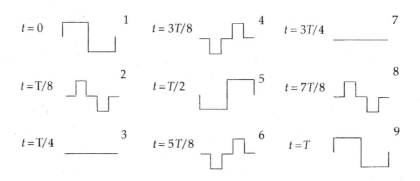

FIGURE 7-15   Motion of the square wave of Figure 7-9 with time. We show the shape at various times within the repeat time T. Note that in the case of the antisymmetric square wave, the repeat time is the period of the second harmonic.

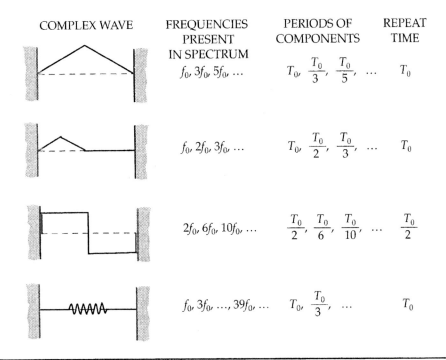

COMPLEX WAVE	FREQUENCIES PRESENT IN SPECTRUM	PERIODS OF COMPONENTS	REPEAT TIME
	$f_0, 3f_0, 5f_0, \ldots$	$T_0, \dfrac{T_0}{3}, \dfrac{T_0}{5}, \ldots$	T_0
	$f_0, 2f_0, 3f_0, \ldots$	$T_0, \dfrac{T_0}{2}, \dfrac{T_0}{3}, \ldots$	T_0
	$2f_0, 6f_0, 10f_0, \ldots$	$\dfrac{T_0}{2}, \dfrac{T_0}{6}, \dfrac{T_0}{10}, \ldots$	$\dfrac{T_0}{2}$
	$f_0, 3f_0, \ldots, 39f_0, \ldots$	$T_0, \dfrac{T_0}{3}, \ldots$	T_0

FIGURE 7-16 The wave shapes studied so far in this chapter with the frequencies of the spectrum, their periods, and their repeat times.

There is a single rule for computing the repeat time and the repeat frequency of any complex wave: **The repeat frequency is the largest common factor of all the frequencies present in the spectrum.** The repeat time is the inverse of this repeat frequency.

Example: What is the largest common factor of the numbers 10, 20, 30? Of 20, 25, 30? Of 60, 62, 64, 66?

Solution: The quantity wanted is the biggest number that divides evenly into all the numbers listed. The numbers 10, 20, and 30 are all multiples of 10, with $10 = 1 \times 10$, $20 = 2 \times 10$, and $30 = 3 \times 10$. The largest common factor of 20, 25, and 30 is 5. The largest common factor of 60, 62, 64, and 66 is 2, since there is no larger number of which all three numbers are integral multiples.

The discussion in this chapter has been illustrated by standing wave examples, but the above rule of repeat times also applies to oscillatory complex traveling waves. The complex traveling waves of Section 6-C contain frequencies of 200 Hz and 400 Hz. The largest common factor is 200 Hz, and the repeat time is 1/200 s in each case.

In each of the previous examples, the repeat time of the complex wave is equal to the period of a mode actually present in the frequency spectrum. However, situations can exist for which the repeat frequency of the complex wave is not equal to any frequency appearing in the frequency spectrum. Our rule fits these cases as well. An example of this is shown in Figure 7-17. This complex wave has been constructed by adding the fourth and the sixth harmonics only ($4f_0$ and $6f_0$). The corresponding frequency spectrum is shown Figure 7-18. According to our rule, the largest

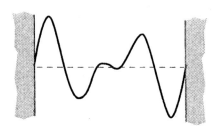

FIGURE 7-17 A complex standing wave formed by adding the fourth and sixth harmonic modes.

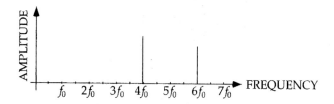

FIGURE 7-18   The frequency spectrum of the standing wave in Figure 7-17.

common factor of the two frequencies is $2f_0$, and the wave should repeat itself after the corresponding period, namely $T_0/2$. The fourth harmonic has a period of $T_0/4$, and will repeat itself every $T_0/4$, while the sixth harmonic has a period of $T_0/6$. Lining up the set of times corresponding to an integer number of cycles for each wave, as in Figure 7-19 may help show why the repeat time is $T_0/2$.

After time $T_0/2$, the fourth mode has gone through two complete cycles, while the sixth mode has gone through three complete cycles. In this example, the repeat frequency is different from that of either of the two modes that make up the complex wave. Nevertheless, our rule holds; $T_0/2$ is still the repeat frequency because it is the largest common factor.

The sound wave emanating from the string of Figure 7-17 would have the same frequency spectrum as shown in Figure 7-18 and would have a perceived pitch corresponding to the frequency $2 f_0$ because the repeat time is $T_0/2$, despite the fact the frequency component $2 f_0$ is missing from the spectrum.

Example: Three traveling waves, A, B, and C, have these component frequencies:

A: 10, 20, 30, and 40 Hz
B: 5, 6, 10, and 12 Hz
C: 6, 12, and 18 Hz

What are the repeat frequencies of the three waves? The repeat times?

Solution: According to the rule, the repeat frequency of A is 10 Hz, of B, 1 Hz, and of C, 6 Hz. In each case, the answer is the largest common factor of the components present. The repeat times are inverses of the frequencies: A is 0.1 s, B, 1 s, and C, 1/6 s.

In example A, the largest common factor is 10 Hz, and this is the repeat frequency. But note that, if the wave is a standing wave, the fundamental frequency might be 10 Hz with first, second, third, and fourth harmonics present; or it might be 5 Hz with all the odd harmonics missing; or some other possibility. The problem does not tell us what the fundamental is, and we do not need to know what the real fundamental is to determine the repeat frequency. Indeed, if the wave is a traveling wave, there are no boundaries and there is no real fundamental frequency at all. Nevertheless, the wave repeats with a repeat frequency of 10 Hz.

❋ *Answer This*

What is the repeat time of a complex wave made up by adding together three sinusoidal waves having frequencies 18 Hz, 24 Hz, and 60 Hz?

7-E. Filters

A **filter** is a device that allows only certain sinusoidal frequency components to pass through and suppresses any others. Filters are used extensively in the transmission of sound waves. Usually, a filter is applied to a sound wave after the wave has been con-

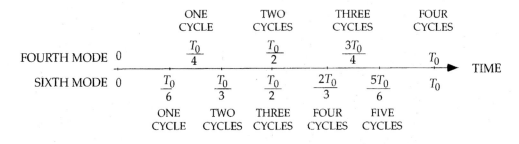

FIGURE 7-19   A chart showing how the fourth and sixth modes repeat simultaneously every half period of the fundamental mode. In that time, the fourth mode has undergone two complete cycles and the sixth, has undergone three complete cycles. There is no shorter time when both modes are together.

verted to an electrical signal by a microphone. The filtered electrical signal may then be converted back to sound by a loudspeaker.

A commonly used filter is called a **bandpass filter**; this filter allows only a certain range of frequencies through and suppresses all others. The **bandwidth** of a filter gives the range of frequencies it will pass. As an example, consider a wave whose repeat frequency is 100 Hz and that has only three odd harmonics, namely 100, 300, and 500 Hz. If this wave is electronically passed through a bandpass filter that allows through only frequencies in the range 400 to 600 Hz (the bandwidth is 600 Hz – 400 Hz = 200 Hz), then only the fifth harmonic, at 500 Hz, will emerge from the filter. However, if the bandwidth is only 50 Hz, so that the bandpass filter only allows frequencies 400 to 450 Hz through, then nothing will get through the filter. A set of different bandpass filters can be used to determine the entire spectrum.

An **electronic frequency spectrum analyzer** is a device that uses such bandpass filters to decompose a complex wave into its Fourier frequency components. The frequency spectrum analyzer then displays the amplitudes of the various component waves. Most modern frequency spectrum analyzers use computers working on digitized sound signals. These produce a frequency spectrum by purely mathematical means rather than by electronic filters.

Another type of filter is the **highpass filter**, which allows through only those frequencies above a certain threshold. For example, a so-called rumble filter in a stereo system is a highpass filter that permits through only frequencies above 80 Hz or so, and thus reduces the annoying low frequencies produced by a turntable drive system. CD players have reduced the need for such filters.

Lowpass filters, on the other hand, let through only those frequencies below a certain threshold. The telephone is a good example of a lowpass filter. For economic reasons, the telephone system is designed to transmit only frequencies below about 3000 Hz. This explains why people's voices sound slightly different on the telephone than in person and also why certain sounds (e.g., [f] and [s]) are difficult to distinguish on the phone. Even though your voice is altered by the telephone, it is still possible to identify the speaker and understand words. When we're spelling an unusual word we might have to resort to saying "f as in Frank, s as in Sam," or the like. Research shows that most conversation is still understandable even when the transmission of only those frequencies below 1800 Hz is allowed. What is equally remark-

able is that conversations passed through a highpass filter allowing only frequencies above 1800 Hz are also understandable. There is clearly a large amount of redundancy in speech information transfer.

The human ear is a bandpass filter to sound, capable of hearing frequencies in the range of 20 Hz to 20,000 Hz. It is probably fortunate that we don't hear lower frequencies, since it might be annoying to hear one's heart beating and blood flowing.

The vocal tract of the human voice can also be thought of as a filter since it damps out certain nonresonant frequencies arising from the vocal folds, while amplifying others near its resonant frequencies. This phenomenon will be discussed in the next chapter. Such a statement about filtering and resonating holds for many musical instruments as well. The violin string is the source of sound that is resonated and filtered by the wooden body of the violin.

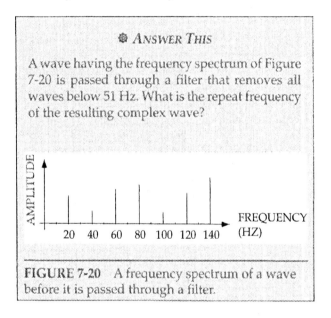

❀ Answer This

A wave having the frequency spectrum of Figure 7-20 is passed through a filter that removes all waves below 51 Hz. What is the repeat frequency of the resulting complex wave?

FIGURE 7-20 A frequency spectrum of a wave before it is passed through a filter.

7-F. Fourier Analysis of Traveling Waves

Thus far, our discussion of Fourier analysis has focused on standing waves. The application of Fourier's theorem to traveling waves is straightforward. If a traveling wave has the same shape as one of the standing complex waves analyzed above, it must contain the same harmonics with the same amplitudes. A difference between standing and traveling waves is that standing waves are subject to boundary conditions, while traveling waves are not. The presence of boundary conditions restricts the set

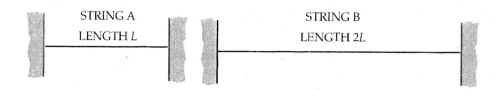

FIGURE 7-21   Two strings, one twice the length of the other. The harmonic series of B has frequencies that are half those of A. For A, the fundamental frequency is $f_{0A} = v/2L$; the harmonic series is $f_{0A}, 2f_{0A}, 3f_{0A}, \ldots$. For B, the fundamental frequency is $f_{0B} = v/4L$; the harmonic series is $f_{0B}, 2f_{0B}, 3f_{0B}, \ldots$.

of frequencies needed to build up a complex wave. A standing complex wave of a certain shape is made up of sinusoidal standing wave components that fit the boundary conditions; the traveling complex wave of the same shape is made up of the same frequencies and amplitudes of sinusoidal traveling waves.

One way to appreciate the differences in the Fourier description of standing and traveling waves is to examine the dependence of the normal mode frequencies upon the length of the medium. Consider two strings, A and B, under the same tension and having equivalent mass densities, so that the propagation velocity is the same in both strings. Both strings will be tied at their ends. However, the lengths of the two strings will be different, one having length L and the other $2L$. The normal modes of these two strings will form different harmonic series. The two strings are shown in Figure 7-21 and their corresponding normal modes are given in the caption (f_{0A} means the fundamental frequency of string A). Because the frequencies of B have an extra factor of 2 in the denominator, then $f_{0B} = (f_{0A})/2$. A scaled chart of the harmonic series of these two strings along a frequency axis looks like Figure 7-22.

Note that the density of frequencies for string B is twice that for string A (that is, the number of frequencies in a given frequency interval for string B is twice that for string A). Since the fundamental frequency of string B is one-half that of string A, the repeat time of an arbitrary complex wave that contains the fundamental as one of its components is twice as long for string B as for string A.

To be a bit more specific, suppose that an impul-

sive wave, such as the one in Figure 7-23, is placed on string A. Since this complex wave is symmetric, it would be expected to contain the fundamental as one of its Fourier components. The repeat time T_A of the complex wave is the period of the fundamental, or $T_A = 1/f_{0A} = 2L/v$. The frequency spectrum is shown at the top right of Figure 7-23. Now suppose that a similar pulse is placed on string B with its accompanying frequency spectrum, also shown in Figure 7-23. As you can see from the frequency spectra of the pulses on strings A and B, the number of normal mode frequencies per unit length along the frequency axis increases as the length of the string increases. Since string B is twice as long as string A, the density of the normal mode frequencies is twice as great.

The repeat time for the pulse on string B would be $T_B = 1/f_{0B} = 2T_A$. The same complex wave on string B has twice the repeat time as it has on string A.

You can think of either repeat time as follows: When the plucked pulse is let go at $t = 0$, its time variation results in two smaller pulses as shown in Figure 7-24 (compare with the discussion of Figure 7-15), which travel one in each direction. A pulse on A must travel from the center as shown with wave velocity v, to one end, a distance $L/2$, then reflect upside down, travel back a distance L to the other end, reflect rightside up, and go $L/2$ to return to the center, where the shape repeats. The total distance traveled on A to repeat is $2L$. Since $v = 2L/T$ where T is the repeat time, then $T_A = 2L/v$, which agrees with our previous calculation as the inverse of the fundamental frequency. The total distance traveled on B is $4L$, which is twice as far, so it takes twice as long.

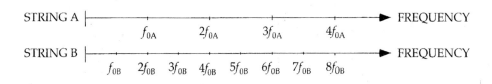

FIGURE 7-22   Comparison of the two harmonic series for strings A and B of Figure 7-21. String B harmonics occur twice as densely as those of string A.

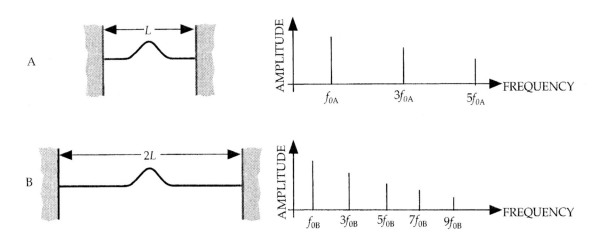

FIGURE 7-23 Impulsive waves on the strings A and B and the corresponding frequency spectra. The impulsive wave is symmetric and contains the odd harmonics. In each frequency spectrum, only a limited number of the components are shown, since the higher harmonics are off-scale. The spectrum of the wave on string B is twice as dense as that on string A.

Next suppose that we place the same pulse as above on a very, very long string. The gap between successive normal mode frequencies becomes exceedingly small, and the frequency of the fundamental approaches 0. In the limiting case of an infinitely long string, any frequency is permissible, not just certain ones as with finite strings. For the infinitely long string, the repeat time would be infinitely long because, when the fundamental frequency becomes a very small number (approaches zero), we take the reciprocal of a very small number, which is very large (1/0 is infinite). An infinitely long repeat time means that the wave never repeats itself. This result is sensi-

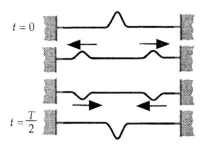

FIGURE 7-24 The time variation of an impulsive wave started on a string results in two smaller waves that travel in opposite directions, reflect, and meet again after a half cycle, *T*, of the fundamental. The process continues with the little pulses reflecting once more and meeting right-side-up after a full period of the fundamental. Each little pulse travels twice the length of the string during this time.

ble, because if the string is infinitely long, the two smaller pulses traveling in opposite directions, which interfere to create the large pulse, never reach the ends of the string, and hence they cannot reflect back, interfere, and repeat the original pulse.

As the medium gets longer and longer, the number of frequencies needed to describe an arbitrary impulsive wave form increases, and the difference between adjacent frequencies decreases. Therefore, to describe an impulsive wave propagating through an infinite medium would require a **continuous frequency spectrum**, as opposed to the **discrete frequency spectrum** we have been considering for periodic waves. Examples of continuous and discrete frequency spectra are provided Figure 7-25.

In practical terms, the propagation of sound through air in any reasonably sized room can be approximated as waves propagating through an infinite medium. If we speak outdoors, it should be obvious that we are in an infinite medium (the air) as long as there is not an obstacle in the way that reflects sound waves. In a small, hollow room, sound can be reflected from the walls, giving rise to standing waves, and in those cases we indeed hear reverberations. Technically, to analyze sound created in an enclosed room would require normal mode frequencies. Realistically, however, in a typical room there is so much sound absorption that no appreciable reflection occurs. This means that the traveling waves are not subject to boundary conditions, and this situation resembles the infinite medium case in the sense that all frequencies are needed to describe arbitrary sound waves.

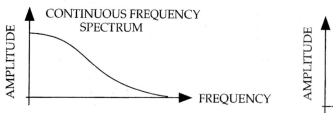
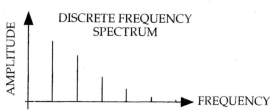

FIGURE 7-25   A continuous spectrum and a discrete spectrum. The discrete spectrum applies to a repeating wave such as a pulse wave on a string of fixed length, while the continuous spectrum applies to a wave that never repeats, such as a pulse wave on a string that is infinitely long.

Two important observations should be highlighted: First, although in the infinite medium case all frequencies are allowed, they need not all be present in the frequency spectrum of a complex wave. For example, one can construct a complex oscillatory traveling wave, and it has a discrete spectrum, because it repeats. Second, there is a general relationship between the number of constituent frequencies needed to construct an impulsive wave by Fourier's theorem and the sharpness of the pulse. The sharper the pulse (the more pointed it is), the more spread out the frequency spectrum, as shown in Figure 7-26. To make the wave narrower, one has to arrange component frequencies to cancel out more of wave in the sides. It takes more high-frequency components to do this canceling out, and the frequency spectrum is therefore broader.

Some additional examples might help clarify the two statements in the previous paragraph. Consider a traveling wave that consists of a series of regularly spaced pulses, with all pulses having the same shape. If the number of pulses is decreased until there is only one, the frequency spectrum will change as shown in Figure 7-27. As the spacing between the pulses increases, the number of frequencies needed to construct the wave increases (i.e., the frequency spectrum becomes more dense, just as when we increased the

length of the string in Figure 7-24). If the spacing between the pulses becomes so large that, for all practical purposes, we have only one pulse that never repeats, we would need a continuous frequency spectrum (i.e., all frequencies are needed) to make up the wave by Fourier's theorem. The dashed line in the first two frequency spectra in Figure 7-27 is called the **envelope**. Note that the envelope remains the same for all three examples in Figure 7-27 because **its shape** depends only on the shape of an individual pulse. However, if we change the shape of the pulses in the complex wave, say, by broadening them, the envelope of the frequency spectrum would fall at a steeper rate.

❀ ANSWER THIS

Figure 7-28 shows a pressure-time graph of a repetitive traveling sound wave. Which of the accompanying plots is the most likely frequency spectrum for this wave? (Hint: Symmetry plays no role here because this is a time graph. Our symmetry arguments apply only to standing waves shown as a function of position.)

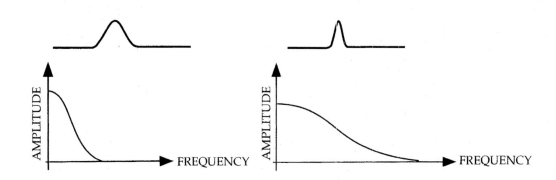

FIGURE 7-26   The relationship between sharpness of an impulsive wave and the spread of the frequency spectrum. The narrower the pulse, the broader the frequency spectrum.

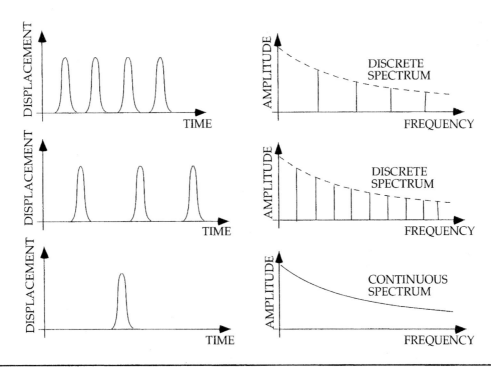

FIGURE 7-27   Pulse waves and their corresponding frequency spectra. The top two pulse waves are repetitive and have discrete spectra. The bottom pulse does not repeat. When the repeat time is longer, the discrete frequency spectrum becomes more dense. In the limit where the pulse never repeats, the spectrum is continuous rather than discrete. The envelope of the spectrum (dotted line in the top two spectra) arises from the shape of a single pulse and remains approximately the same.

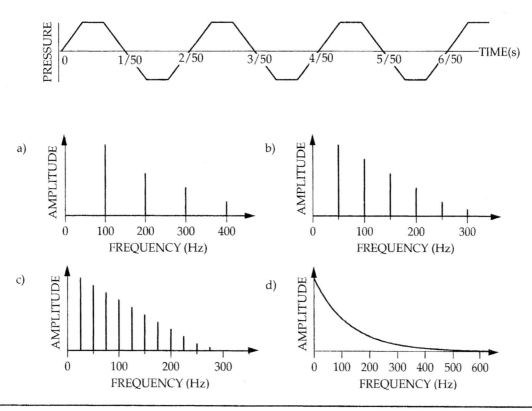

FIGURE 7-28   A pressure-time graph for a sound wave at top. Which of the frequency spectra is appropriate for it?

Exercises

1. Draw the frequency spectrum of a pure tone sound wave of 100 Hz.

2. What is the repeat time of the wave shown in Figure 7-29?

   a) 1/100 s
   b) 2/100 s
   c) 3/100 s
   d) 6/100 s
   e) none of these

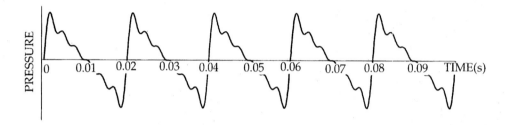

FIGURE 7-29   Pressure-time graph of a traveling sound wave. The wave is made up of a harmonic series containing many frequencies.

3. What is the frequency of the fundamental in the harmonic series making up the wave in Figure 7-29?

   a) 20 Hz
   b) 50 Hz
   c) 100 Hz
   d) 250 Hz
   e) not possible to tell from the information given

4. Assume that the relative amplitudes of the harmonics of the wave in Figure 7-29 are 1, 1/2, 1/3, 1/4, 1/5, etc. (or, in decimal form, 1, 0.5, 0.33, 0.25, 0.20, 0.17, etc.). Draw a plot of the frequency spectrum.

5. Suppose a bandpass filter removes all frequencies in the spectrum of the wave in Figure 7-29 except frequencies in the range 145 to 355 Hz. What frequencies make up the resulting wave that passes through the filter?

   a) 150, 200, 250, 300, 350 Hz
   b) 200, 300 Hz
   c) 145, 200, 250, 350, 355 Hz
   d) 145, 150, 155, . . . 350, 355 Hz
   e) none of these sets

6. What is the repeat time of the filtered wave in question 5?

   a) 1/100 s
   b) 1/50 s
   c) 1/150 s
   d) 1/145 s
   e) none of these

7. At time $t = 0$, the standing wave shown in Figure 7-30 is set up on a string. The string has length of 5 ft and wave velocity 50 ft/s. What are the frequencies of the first eight allowed normal modes on this string?

a) $2.5, 5.0, 7.5, \ldots, 17.5, 20.0$ Hz

b) $2.5, 7.5, 12.5, \ldots, 32.5, 37.5$ Hz

c) $5, 10, 15, \ldots, 35, 40$ Hz

d) $5, 15, 25, \ldots, 65, 75$ Hz

e) $10, 20, 30, \ldots, 80$ Hz

8. Is the complex wave shown at $t = 0$ in Figure 7-30 symmetric, antisymmetric, or of mixed symmetry?

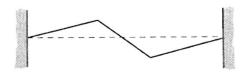

FIGURE 7-30 Wave shape on a string tied at both ends at time $t = 0$. The length of the string is $L = 5$ ft. The propagation velocity of waves on the string is $v = 50$ ft/s.

9. According to Fourier's theorem, which of the frequencies in Question 7 will you *likely* need to add to make up the complex wave of Figure 7-30?

a) $2.5, 5.0, 7.5, \ldots,$ Hz

b) $2.5, 7.5, 12.5, \ldots,$ Hz

c) $5, 10, 15, \ldots,$ Hz

d) $5, 15, 25, \ldots,$ Hz

e) $10, 20, 30, \ldots,$ Hz

10. Suppose that, in order of increasing frequency, the relative amplitudes of the first four constituent sinusoidal components of the wave of Figure 7-30 are 1, 0.5, 0.3, and 0.1. Plot a frequency spectrum for the complex wave.

11. Redo Question 7, assuming that the length of the string is now $L = 10$ ft. and everything else is the same. The answer set given in 7 will still apply.

12. Redo Question 9 if everything is the same except the length of the string, which is now $L = 10$ ft. The answer set given in 9 will still apply.

13. Redo Question 10 if everything is the same except that the length of the string is now $L = 10$ ft. Put the frequency spectrum on the same sheet of paper as that of Question 10. Explain as precisely as you can what happens to the frequency spectrum of the complex standing wave of Figure 7-30 as you increase the length of the string.

14. Do the same operations as in Questions 7 through 10 for the standing complex wave shown in Figure 7-31, except now use the values, 0.2, 1, 0.4, and 0.2 for the amplitudes of the first four constituent frequencies needed in Question 10. With regard to the frequency spectrum of this second complex wave, can you think of a reason why the relative amplitude of the second constituent sinusoidal wave is larger than the relative amplitudes of the other constituent sinusoidal waves?

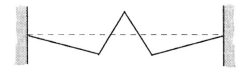

FIGURE 7-31 A different standing wave at $t = 0$ on the string in Figure 7-30. The properties of the string are the same as in that figure.

15. A standing wave on a string is shown in Figure 7-32 at one instance of time. You can say that the wave

    a) is symmetric
    b) is antisymmetric
    c) has mixed symmetry
    d) is none of these

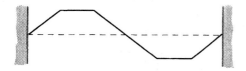

FIGURE 7-32 A wave shape on a string tied at both ends at $t = 0$.

16. If the fundamental frequency for standing waves on the string of Figure 7-32 is 10 Hz, which of the frequency spectra in Figure 7-33 is most likely for the wave shape shown in that figure?

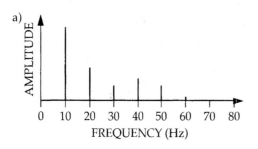

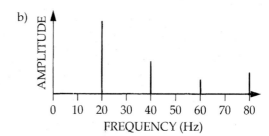

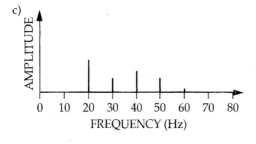

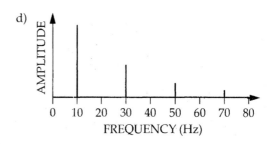

FIGURE 7-33 Frequency spectra choices for question 16.

17. A string tied at both ends has a fundamental frequency of 10 Hz. How long would you have to wait until the string, as it vibrates starting from the shape shown in Figure 7-32, has the shape shown in Figure 7-34?

    a) 1/5 s   b) 1/10 s   c) 1/20 s   d) 1/40 s   e) 1/80 s

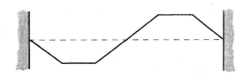

FIGURE 7-34 The wave in Figure 7-32 at a later time.

18. Match the pressure-time graphs on the left of Figure 7-35 with the appropriate frequency spectra on the right.

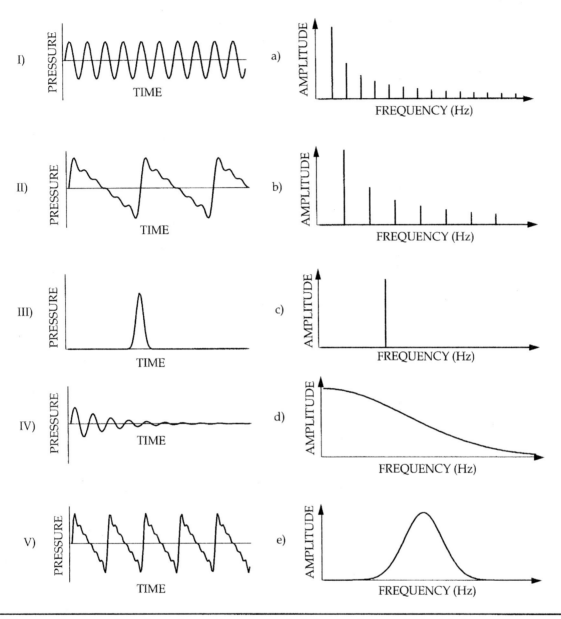

FIGURE 7-35 Pressure-time plots of sound waves on the left are to be matched with the appropriate frequency spectra on the right.

19. Match the pressure-time graphs on the left of Figure 7-36 with the appropriate frequency spectra on the right.

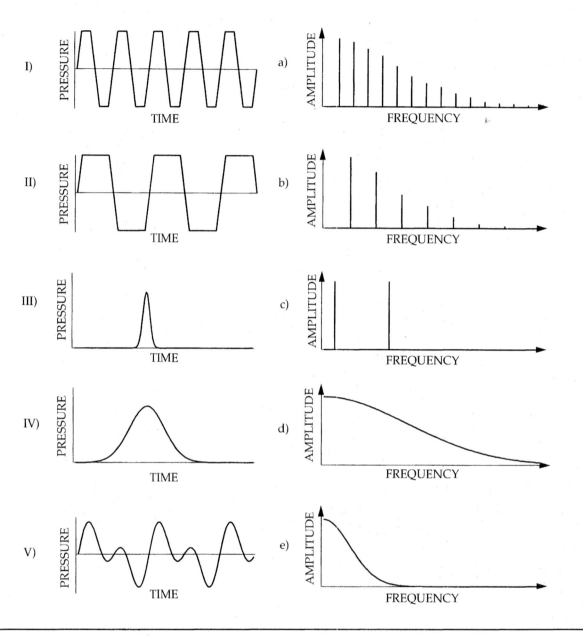

FIGURE 7-36   Pressure-time plots of sound waves to be matched with the appropriate frequency spectra on the right.

8
Speech Production

Up to this point, we have studied the physics of waves, including topics such as traveling and standing waves of both the sinusoidal and complex variety, resonance, and Fourier analysis. Finally, we are ready to apply all of our physics knowledge to various topics, such as speech production, speech analysis, and speech recognition. This chapter deals with speech production and speech analysis (spectrograms) in general. The next chapter covers analysis of specific speech sounds.

8-A. *Vocal Organs*

The vocal organs are the parts of our anatomy used to produce speech. They include the lungs, the trachea (windpipe), the larynx (which contains the vocal folds), the pharynx (throat), the nasal cavity (nose), and the oral cavity (mouth). These organs form a tube starting at the lungs and ending at the lips.

The vocal tract is the part of this tube lying above the larynx. It consists of the pharynx, mouth, and nose, as shown in Figure 8-1. In adult humans, the oral cavity forms a right angle with the throat, with only the epiglottis (which folds down as needed) and the vocal cords preventing food from entering the lungs. In great apes and infants, there is a gentle curve from the oral cavity to the throat, and the soft palate hangs lower in the back of the oral cavity. Also, the tongue fills up even more of the oral cavity and sits much farther back, helping guide liquids and food into the esophagus. These structural differences put adult humans at greater risk of choking than great apes or infants, but make it possible for us to produce speech as we do. The nasal cavity is actually much bigger than the oral cavity. We will make use of this fact when we talk about the production of nasal sounds in Chapter 9. The shape of the vocal tract can be varied with the help of our tongue, lips, and soft palate (and, in some languages, the cheeks and/or the pharyngeal muscles). By changing the shape of the vocal tract, we are able to produce different sounds.

The mechanism for producing speech proceeds as follows. The vocal folds vibrate, thereby producing a pressure pulse containing many frequencies—in fact, the frequencies form a harmonic series, f_0, $2f_0$, $3f_0$, $4f_0$, ..., of the type we have studied. These frequencies enter the air tube in the vocal tract, but the air tube resonates only at its natural frequencies of vibration (F_1, F_2, F_3, F_4, ...). This means that some of the frequencies contained in the pulse created by the vocal folds are enhanced while others are damped. Thus, the vibrations are analogous to the normal modes of an air column that is closed at one end (the larynx) and open at the other (the lips). We will show how closely this air column is an analog of the vocal tract a little later. Let us now begin from the beginning and build our knowledge of speech production one step at a time.

8-B. *Vocal Fold Vibration*

The energy that goes into making speech sounds originates in the muscles of the chest and abdomen. These muscles force air out from the lungs, and this air sets the vocal folds vibrating.

The **vocal folds** (or cords) are folds of ligament that extend from the Adam's apple at the front of the larynx to the **arytenoid cartilages** at the back. They are often called **vocal cords**. By using the laryngeal muscles, the vocal folds can be brought together so that they shut off the air passage from the lungs.

The space between the vocal folds is called the **glottis**, and the air pulses created by the vocal folds are called **glottal pulses**. Glottal pulses are produced

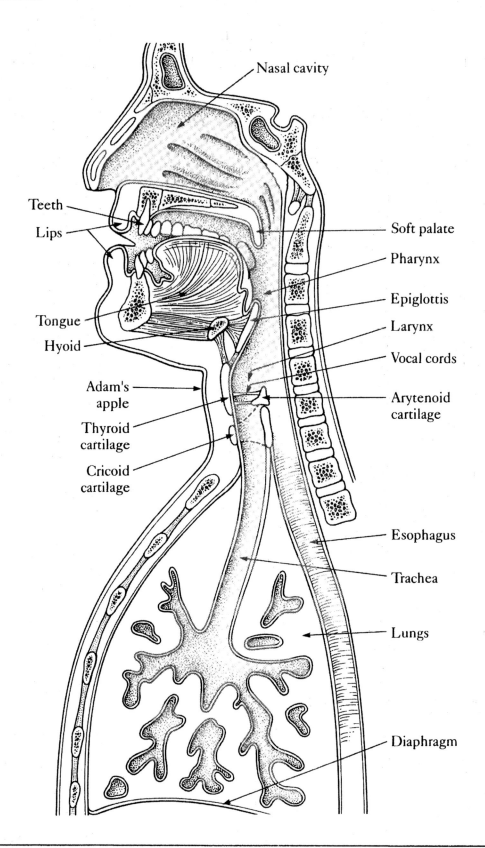

FIGURE 8-1 The human vocal organs. From: *The Speech Chain* by Peter B. Denes and Elliot N. Pinson © by W. H. Freeman and Company. Used with permission of Worth Publishers.

at very regular intervals. The repeating, periodic wave that results from vocal fold vibrations is called the **glottal wave**.

The mechanism by which the vocal folds vibrate is as follows. Assume that the vocal folds are initially closed. As a stream of air from the lungs enters the trachea, air pressure builds up below the vocal folds. When this air pressure reaches a certain level, the muscles holding the vocal folds together give way, and the vocal folds are literally blown apart. This coming apart of the vocal folds serves to release the excess pressure, thereby creating a pressure pulse. As soon as the excess pressure is released, the vocal folds return to their closed position due to the reduced pressure of the flowing air, and the cycle begins again.

You might think that, once the vocal folds get blown apart and the air from the lungs starts rushing through, there would be little chance of shutting the cords back up again against the flow of air. It actually is quite easy to close them because of the **Bernoulli effect:** The sudden rush of air in the trachea results in a drop in pressure, and thus there is a sucking effect that tends to pull the vocal folds back together again. The Bernoulli effect is what causes a baseball to curve, an airplane to stay in the sky, and a shower curtain to be sucked into a shower stall. We need a bit more physics background to delve into this effect in detail, so we won't do so here.

Thus, the vocal folds are blown apart by the air pressure that builds up beneath them, then sucked back together by the low pressure created as the air rushes by. Once they are closed, the air pressure builds up again, and the cycle repeats itself. The opening and closing of the vocal folds creates a sequence of air puffs. The frequency of these air puffs varies from individual to individual, ranging from 60 to 500 cycles per second. For men, the average frequency with which the vocal folds open and shut is about 120 Hz. It is about 225 Hz for a woman and about 265 Hz for a child. Those are high frequencies. The vocal folds get blown apart and come back together over 200 times each second for a typical woman.

Recall that the fundamental frequency of vibration of a string of length L with wave velocity v is $v/2L$ and thus depends on the length of the string and the propagation velocity. The propagation velocity in turn depends on the mass density and the tension of the string. Similarly, the exact frequency of vibration of the vocal folds depends on their length and propagation velocity. Their propagation velocity depends on the mass and tension of the vocal folds. Short, small, or tightly stretched vocal folds vibrate at a high frequency, resulting in a high-pitched voice. Long, massive, or very lax vocal folds vibrate at a low frequency, resulting in a deep voice. Men, who have more massive vocal folds, have lower pitched voices than women and children, but by adjusting the tension in our vocal folds (e.g., by tightening them to sing a high note) we all have some control over the pitch of our voices.

As stated earlier, the wave generated by the opening and closing of the vocal folds is periodic. Figure 8-2 is an approximation of this pressure wave. The glottal wave drawn in this figure has a repeat time of .008 seconds and thus has a repeat frequency of $f_0 = 1/.008 = 125$ Hz. This repeat frequency will be the fundamental frequency in the harmonic series that could be used to construct the traveling glottal wave by Fourier's theorem. Thus, the harmonic series of

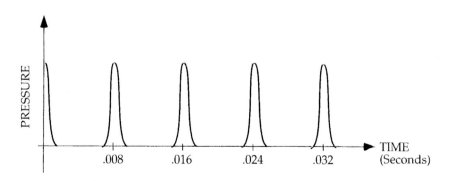

FIGURE 8-2   Approximate shape of the glottal wave for a person with a fundamental frequency of 125 Hz.

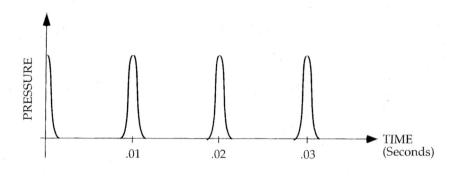

FIGURE 8-3   Approximate shape of the glottal wave for a person with a fundamental frequency of 100 Hz.

this glottal wave is 125 Hz, 250 Hz, 375 Hz, 500 Hz, . . . The pitch we associate with a person's voice corresponds to the lowest frequency of the glottal harmonic series. For the glottal wave in Figure 8-2, we would hear a pitch of about 125 Hz, which means that the wave was likely produced by a male speaker.

A different person might produce the glottal wave shown in Figure 8-3. This glottal wave has a repeat time of .01 second, and thus its repeat frequency is f_0 = 100 Hz (this person has a deeper voice than the one whose glottal wave is shown in Figure 8-2). That means that the glottal wave of this speaker has a harmonic series equal to 100 Hz, 200 Hz, 300 Hz, 400 Hz, ... The frequency spectra of the glottal waves in Figures 8-2 and 8-3 can be approximated by the graphs in Figures 8-4 and 8-5.

Notice a few features of these two frequency spectra. First, both frequency spectra have the same **envelope curve** (shown as a dashed line), the reason being that the shape of each individual glottal pulse is the same in Figures 8-2 and 8-3. Also notice that the spacing between the frequency components of the frequency spectrum of Figure 8-4 is wider than the spacing between the frequency components of the frequency spectrum of Figure 8-5. The reason is that

the harmonic series of the glottal pulse in Figure 8-2 is 125 Hz, 250 Hz, 375 Hz, 500 Hz, . . . , while that of the glottal pulse in Figure 8-3 is 100 Hz, 200 Hz, 300 Hz, 400 Hz, ... Thus, the gap between any two adjacent frequency components in the frequency spectrum of Figure 8-2 is 125 Hz, while the gap between any two adjacent frequency components in the frequency spectrum of Figure 8-3 is 100 Hz. This should not be surprising if you look back at Figure 7-27 in Chapter 7, since some of these figures show complex waves and their corresponding frequency spectra that are very similar to the two glottal waves drawn in Figures 8-2 and 8-3.

We now know that the glottal wave produced by the vocal folds is periodic, and we also know the general shape of this complex pressure wave. We know what its frequency spectrum looks like. Yet, we never actually hear what this glottal wave sounds like. The reason is that it must pass through the vocal tract and, as we shall see shortly, the vocal tract modifies the glottal wave, enhancing those frequencies that correspond to the vocal tract's natural resonant frequencies, and damping those that do not. We might understand this phenomenon better by making an analogy between speaking and playing a trumpet.

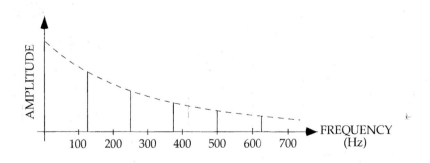

FIGURE 8-4   Frequency spectrum of the glottal wave in Figure 8-2.

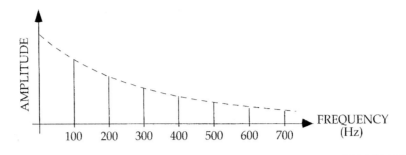

FIGURE 8-5   Frequency spectrum of the glottal wave in Figure 8-3.

When somebody is playing a trumpet, we don't hear the buzzing noise made by the lips at the mouthpiece of the trumpet; we only hear what this buzzing sounds like after it gets modified by the air tract of the trumpet. There is one important difference between playing a trumpet and speaking; the trumpet player could remove the trumpet from his or her lips and buzz the lips so that we could hear the unmodified sound made by the vibrating lips. We cannot rip out our vocal folds and vibrate them to hear their unmodified sound. However, people whose larynxes have been removed due to cancer hold artificial larynxes, buzzers that vibrate at an appropriate frequency, next to their throats to simulate the glottal sound and set up vibrations in their vocal tracts that can be shaped into fairly intelligible speech by the articulators.

In summary, the glottal wave does not convey any linguistic information; it is not directly responsible for making a sound that we would recognize as, say, the vowel [i] as in "bee". The glottal wave is only the source of the frequencies whose amplitudes get enhanced or damped by the vocal tract. The shape of the vocal tract differentiates the speech sounds that we recognize as particular vowels or consonants.

8-C. Acoustic Properties of the Vocal Tract

The vocal tract acts as a resonant cavity that selects out certain frequencies in the glottal wave for amplification. For the moment, we will restrict ourselves to discussing the mechanism by which we use our vocal tract to articulate vowels. Let us begin by considering some facts we know about speech sounds. Different vowels sound different; we have no difficulty hearing distinctly different sounds for the vowels in the mid-

dle of the words "head" ([ɛ]) and "hood" ([ʊ]). (Appendix B includes a list of the phonetic symbols used in this book.) Further, we can recognize a vowel even when it is articulated at different pitches; we recognize the [ʊ] in "hood" when it is pronounced by a child whose glottal wave has a high-pitched repeat frequency of 350 Hz, as well as when it is pronounced by a man whose glottal wave has a low-pitched repeat frequency of 100 Hz. From this we can conclude that our ability to recognize vowel sounds does not depend on the pitch (the repeat frequency of the glottal wave) at which the vowels are articulated.

To begin to understand how the vocal tract makes different sounds, we could try to model how it might work. As mentioned earlier, we can consider the vocal tract as an air column that is closed at one end (the throat) and open at the other (the lips). Let us use our knowledge of normal modes to compute the first few frequencies of vibration of an air column of the size of our vocal tract. All we need to do is make some estimates of the size of the vocal tract and apply our boundary conditions.

Let us assume that we are going to pronounce the vowel schwa, [ə], as in the beginning of the word "**about**." When we articulate this vowel, we shape our vocal tract into a more or less uniformly shaped air tube. From an anatomy book, we can look up the typical length of the vocal tract, starting from the glottis and ending at the lips (for the moment, we will neglect the nasal cavity, since it is closed by the soft palate when we articulate vowels). The vocal tract is about 17 cm long (6.7 in). The other fact we will need is the speed of sound in air, which we already know is about 335 m/s (1100 ft/s). Recall the boundary conditions that apply to an air column that is open at one end and closed at the other (Section 3-D). A displacement node must be present at the closed end, and a displacement antinode must be present at the open

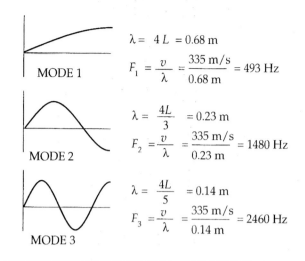

$$\lambda = 4L = 0.68 \text{ m}$$

MODE 1

$$F_1 = \frac{v}{\lambda} = \frac{335 \text{ m/s}}{0.68 \text{ m}} = 493 \text{ Hz}$$

$$\lambda = \frac{4L}{3} = 0.23 \text{ m}$$

$$F_2 = \frac{v}{\lambda} = \frac{335 \text{ m/s}}{0.23 \text{ m}} = 1480 \text{ Hz}$$

MODE 2

$$\lambda = \frac{4L}{5} = 0.14 \text{ m}$$

$$F_3 = \frac{v}{\lambda} = \frac{335 \text{ m/s}}{0.14 \text{ m}} = 2460 \text{ Hz}$$

MODE 3

FIGURE 8-6 Crude model of vocal tract resonances for the neutral vowel [ə]. For this vowel, we assume that the vocal tract is a uniformly shaped air column open at one end and closed at the other.

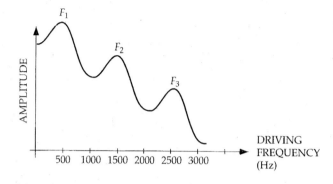

FIGURE 8-7 Frequency response curve for the vowel [ə].

end. The first three modes, along with the corresponding wavelengths and frequencies, are shown in Figure 8-6 (cf. Figure 3-10).

According to our crude model, the first three frequencies at which our vocal tract resonates when pronouncing the vowel [ə] would be approximately 500, 1500, and 2500 Hz. Because the vocal tract enhances certain frequencies as they pass through but suppresses others that don't correspond to allowed wavelengths for the vocal tract tube, it is often referred to as a **filter**. As it turns out, the vocal tract is not a perfect resonator; the sound energy gets damped as it encounters muscle and surface tissue in the vocal tract. The total resonance curve for the vocal tract resulting from our crude model is obtained by overlapping three damped resonance curves of the type shown in Figure 4-3. Thus, the resonance curve for the vocal tract using our model would look like Figure 8-7.

Other names given to the resonance curve are **frequency response curve, filter spectrum,** and **frequency characteristic curve.** What the frequency response curve tells us is that when we drive our vocal tract with our vocal folds, the amplitudes of the frequency components of the resulting sound wave (the frequency spectrum) will be modulated by this frequency response curve. In other words, the frequency response curve will be an estimate of the envelope for the frequency spectrum of the sound we hear, depending on how well the frequencies of the

frequency response curve (the filter frequencies) match the frequencies of the glottal spectrum (the source frequencies).

This interaction between the glottal spectrum (the source of the sound) and the vocal tract (an air tube open at one end that filters the glottal wave frequencies) is modeled in Figure 8-8. Certain frequencies are emitted by the vocal folds depending on their length, mass, and tension, as shown in the spectra on the left in Figure 8-8. The top one is the glottal spectrum for a fundamental frequency of 125 Hz, the lower one for an f_0 of 100 Hz.

As we have discussed, the vocal tract is predisposed to resonate more at certain frequencies depending on its length (and, as we shall see later, its specific shape; for [ə] we don't have to worry about this factor). The frequencies at which the vocal tract will resonate the most are represented by the peaks in the frequency response curves or filter spectra, shown in the middle of Figure 8-8. Since we assume that the vocal tracts of the two speakers are the same length, the two filter spectra (top and bottom) are the same. The fundamental frequency and harmonics of the glottal wave have no effect on the frequency response curve.

Passing through the vocal tract (through the vocal filter) changes the glottal wave on its route to the open air. Thus, the sound that comes out of the mouth has resonances at the harmonics of the glottal source, but each of those harmonics has been enhanced or damped by the vocal tract filter, depending on how well the harmonic frequencies correspond to the resonance curve frequencies.

The two frequency output spectra on the right of Figure 8-8 correspond to the actual sound of the vowel [ə] obtained by applying our model of the vocal tract to two different speakers. The top output

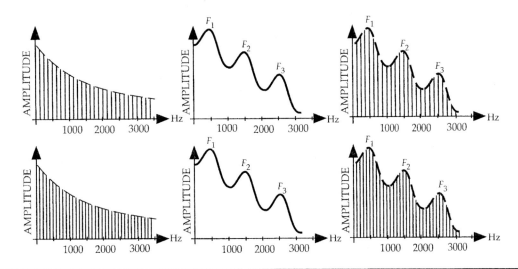

FIGURE 8-8   The frequency spectra (the two plots at the right) of two different speakers pronouncing the vowel [ə]. The glottal frequency (source) spectra (the two plots at the left) are modified by the frequency response curve (filter; middle plots), resulting in the frequency spectra (output) shown at the right.

spectrum has frequencies at wider intervals (is less dense) than the bottom one because it represents a higher fundamental frequency. However, the overall shapes (envelopes) of the two output spectra are the same because both glottal waves were filtered by the same vocal tract.

The relative peaks in the output frequency spectrum of the vowel [ə] shown in Figure 8-8—of which there are three, labeled F_1, F_2, and F_3, at frequencies around 500, 1500, and 2500 Hz—are called **formants**. Formants are the frequencies that are heard most clearly by the listener because they have been resonated by the vocal tract.

In this case, the frequencies of both of these source spectra are close enough together that there is at least a near match with the resonant frequencies of the vocal tract filter. That is, the larynx is providing vibrations at frequencies at which the vocal tract naturally resonates. For this reason, the frequency response curve and the output spectrum look very similar. In the case of a very high-pitched voice, however, there may be a mismatch in the case of some vowels. For example, suppose a vowel had formants at 400 Hz, 1000 Hz, and 2400 Hz, and the speaker's glottal frequency spectrum had a very high f_0 of 400 Hz. The glottal wave would have a harmonic series equal to 400 Hz, 800 Hz, 1200 Hz, 1600 Hz, 2000 Hz, 2400 Hz, 2800 Hz, ... Thus, while there would be a source frequency to match the lowest resonant frequency of the vocal tract at 400 Hz, there would be no 1000 Hz glottal pulse that could be enhanced by the

vocal tract's resonant frequency response, as shown in Figure 8-9.

The 400 Hz and the 2400 Hz glottal harmonic frequencies would be well enhanced at F_1 and F_3 respectively, since they match the resonances at those frequencies. However, the resulting output spectrum would have a very flattened F_2 due to this mismatch; the 800 Hz harmonic would be too low, and the 1200 Hz harmonic would be too high for the 1000 Hz filter format. The vocal cord vibration would not provide any energy at 1000 Hz to be enhanced; the vocal tract cannot enhance frequencies that are not present. Thus, the glottal source spectrum has no influence on the frequency response curve of the vocal tract, but it may affect the intensity or specificity of the output formants that are actually produced if there is a mismatch of this sort between the source and the filter. Fortunately, the human speech perception system is flexible enough that one such piece of missing information is not usually a major problem, unless the utterance is unclear for other reasons as well.

Thus far, we've only considered the vowel schwa, [ə], for which the vocal tract is relatively uniformly shaped—the tongue and lips are basically at rest. The articulatory requirements of other vowels distort the shape of the vocal tract from this relative uniformity. For example, for [ɑ] (as in "bah!"), the jaw is lowered and the tongue is moved back toward the pharynx, widening the mouth opening and narrowing the passage through the pharynx. In contrast, the vowel [u] requires lip rounding (accompanied by lip protru-

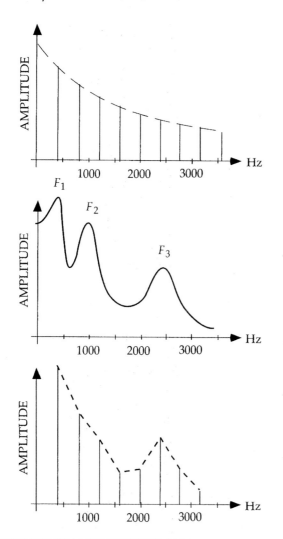

FIGURE 8-9 A glottal pulse based on a harmonic series of 400 Hz is mismatched in the second formant with a vocal tract having resonant frequencies at 400 Hz, 1000 Hz, and 2500 Hz. There is no component in the glottal pulse at 1000 Hz to be resonated at that frequency. The dashed envelope curve is simply a line connecting the amplitudes of the frequencies present.

at 530, 1840, and 2480 Hz for male speakers pronouncing the vowel [ɛ] in "head." This is close to what our model predicted by considering the vocal tract to be an air column 17 cm long open at one end and closed at the other; the vocal tract configuration for [ɛ] is similar to that for [ə]. For a female speaking the [ɛ] sound, the average formants are 610, 2330, and 2990 Hz. On the other hand, for the sound [u] in "who'd" spoken by a male, the average formants are at 300, 870, and 2240 Hz, while for a female they are at 370, 950, and 2670 Hz.

Now we can understand why we are able to recognize vowel sounds spoken by people whose voices vary in pitch (i.e., people with different repeat frequencies of their glottal waves). Although each person's glottal pitch sounds different, each vowel requires distinct shaping of the vocal tract. The shape of the vocal tract influences the frequency response curve, which in turn affects the output **formant structure** (where the formants are and the relative spacing between them). The glottal wave can sharpen or flatten the peaks in the output spectrum, but it cannot change its basic shape. As a result, the output spectrum of every vowel has a distinct pattern, and it is this distinct pattern that we use to recognize the specific vowel sounds. Hence, our ability to recognize vowel sounds is dictated by the shape of the vocal tract, not by the shape of the glottal wave.

It is important to realize that the formant structure of a particular vowel is the result of the shape of the entire vocal tract. It would be a simplification to say that, for example, the back of the vocal tract gave rise to formant F_1 in the vowel in "head" and that the front of the vocal tract gave rise to the formant F_3. Although some portions of the vocal tract may have more influence on some portions of the output wave, each formant depends on the shape of the whole vocal tract.

8-D. Sound Spectrographs

Although we have already learned a great deal about speech production, we are limited if we continue discussing speech production in terms of pressure-time graphs and frequency spectra. The reason is that, during speech, we are continuously changing the shape of our vocal tracts as well as turning our vocal folds on and off depending on whether the sound we want to make is a vowel or a (voiceless) consonant. Thus, what we need is many frequency spectra taken during the course of speech separated by very short time

sion), which has the effect of lengthening the vocal tract tube. Thus, the formants for vowels other than schwa will not be nice, neat multiples of each other.

Researchers have determined the average values for the first three formants for different vowel sounds made by men, women, and children. (Every individual of the same gender has slightly different formants for a given vowel, and averages of the formants need to be taken over many speakers.) One finds formants

intervals. Since a frequency spectrum shows what is happening at some instant in time, taking many frequency spectra as time passes will let us see what a vocal tract is doing to produce speech sounds. The device that is used for this purpose is called the **sound spectrograph**.

The sound spectrograph is a machine that effectively contains a series of bandpass filters of adjoining bandwidths. The way the spectrograph works is fairly easy to understand. As a complex sound wave enters the spectrograph (after being "heard" by a microphone), the different frequency components of the wave are extracted and displayed as a function of time. The spectrograph provides us with a pictorial record of what transpired during speech, called a **spectrogram**. An example is provided in Figure 8-10.

In contrast to a frequency spectrum, which shows frequency on the horizontal axis and amplitude on the vertical axis, on a spectrogram the vertical axis of the spectrogram plots the frequency, while the horizontal axis denotes time. On a spectrogram, a band that is higher up on the spectrogram represents a higher-frequency sound, while a band that is farther to the right represents a sound that was produced later in time. Thus, the horizontal axis of the spectrogram in Figure 8-10 is marked off in milliseconds (ms) and the vertical axis in Hertz (Hz). Using the horizontal axis, we can see that it takes this speaker approximately 2000 ms (2 seconds) to produce the phrase "a tot, a dot." Using the vertical axis, we can identify formants in the first vowel (centered at 169 ms) at approximately 700, 1400, and 2700 Hz.

On a spectrogram, there is no axis available for amplitude. Therefore, the spectrograph draws bands of different darkness, and the darkness of the bands denotes the amplitude of the wave at the particular range of frequencies in question; the darker the band, the more intense the sound. The dark portions of the spectrogram in Figure 8-10 represent the loudest portions of speech—vowel formants and some intense portions of consonants.

Thus, a formant at a certain frequency—that is, a frequency at which the glottal wave has been enhanced by the resonance properties of the vocal tract—will be represented as a relatively narrow, dark, horizontal band. For example, if a typical male is pronouncing a vowel such as [ʌ] in "number" (the stressed counterpart to schwa), the spectrogram will have dark horizontal bands at the formants around frequencies 500, 1500, and 2500 Hz for male speakers. The length of the band (from left to right) will depend on how long the vowel is pronounced. In Figure 8-10,

for example, the first vowel ([ə], the article "a") lasts a shorter time than the second vowel ([ɑ] in "tot") and a much shorter time than the fourth vowel ([ɑ] in "dot").

In contrast, white noise will show up with equal darkness at all frequencies. On a spectrogram, it will look like a scratchy vertical band. The thickness of the band will depend on how long the noise lasts. A sudden, brief noise that ranges over a variety of frequencies, such as a door slam or a stop/plosive consonant (e.g., [p], [t], or [k]), will also appear as a scratchy vertical band, but the scratches will not cover the entire vertical range of the spectrogram, since the noise will not cover all frequencies. A prolonged aperiodic sound, such as the sound of popcorn being shaken or a fricative sound (e.g., [f], [θ], [s], or [ʃ]—"f," voiceless "th," "s," or "sh") will be more spread out horizontally, but will still look undefined (scratchy) both horizontally and vertically. The noise corresponding to the consonant [t] can be seen in Figure 8-10 at approximately 400–500 ms, 840–850 ms, and 1860–1870 ms. This high-frequency noise extends from about 1000 to 4500 Hz, with the loudest portions at the higher frequencies. The first [t] occurs at the beginning of a word and therefore lasts much longer than the other two (because it is more heavily aspirated— more air is released—in that word position).

A spectrogram may be drawn in such a way that more detail is visible with respect to the time dimension (**wide band**) or with respect to the frequency dimension (**narrow band**). If time detail is visible, it will take the form of **vertical striations** within the horizontal energy bands (formants), as can be seen in Figure 8-10, especially during the vowel portion of the last word, "dot." Each of these striations represents one glottal pulse. Obviously, they will only be visible when the vocal folds are vibrating—that is, the sound produced is **voiced** (a vowel or a voiced consonant such as [m], [b], [z], or [w]). Furthermore, they will be very faint where the signal is faint (e.g., between formants). On a wide-band spectrogram such as this, we can count the number of striations per second, and this will correspond directly to the number of cycles per second in the person's fundamental frequency. For example, the fourth vowel (the [ɑ] from the word "dot") on the wide band spectrogram in Figure 8-10 lasts about 260 ms (or 0.26 seconds), and we can pick out about 24 vertical striations in that time. Therefore (because 24 cycles/0.26 s = 108 cycles/s), we can determine that this adult male's fundamental frequency is about 108 cycles per second, or 108 Hz.

If frequency detail is visible, it will take the form

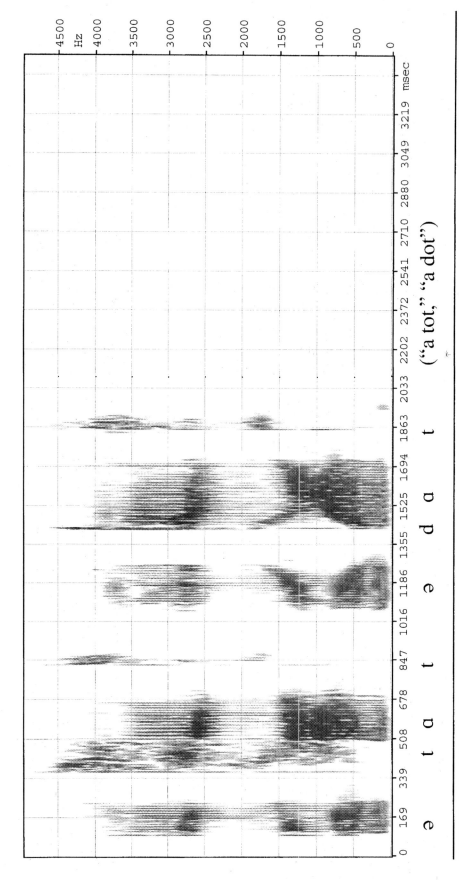

FIGURE 8-10 Wide-band spectrogram of a male saying "A tot, a dot."

of **horizontal striations** within the horizontal energy bands (formants) on a narrow-band spectrogram, as shown in Figure 8-11. Each of these horizontal striations represents one of the enhanced frequencies from the glottal source spectrum. Again, these will be visible only for voiced sounds, and their darkness will be determined by the degree to which that particular harmonic is amplified by the vocal tract. The same utterance depicted in Figure 8-10 is represented in Figure 8-11 as a narrow-band spectrogram. On this narrow-band spectrogram, we can identify 5 (horizontal) harmonics in the fourth vowel in a span of about 520 Hz (counting up from the bottom), indicating that the person's f_0 is about 104 Hz, about the same as we calculated from the wide-band spectrogram. This is as expected, since it is the same utterance produced by the same speaker. (For more precision, a wide-band spectrogram that was more spread out in time—e.g., showing just one word— and a narrow-band spectrogram that was more spread out in frequencies—e.g., showing only 0–1000 Hz—could be used.) Generally, it is easier to calculate fundamental frequencies using a narrow-band spectrogram than using a wide-band one.

For a female speaker saying the same sentence, the vertical striations on the wide-band spectrogram will be closer together (more pulses per second, higher frequency), as shown in Figure 8-12. On the other hand, as we have seen when we discussed frequency spectra, the fundamental glottal pulse and its harmonics are farther apart in terms of frequency for a female speaker. Thus, the horizontal striations on a narrow-band spectrogram will be farther apart for a female speaker than for a male speaker, as shown in Figure 8-13. Even more so than for the male speaker, it's easier to calculate the female speaker's f_0 using the narrow-band spectrogram (about 4 horizontal striations per 1000 Hz, or 250 Hz) than using the wide-band spectrogram.

In addition to being the easiest display to use for determining the speaker's fundamental frequency, the horizontal striations on a narrow-band spectrogram also reveal pitch changes in the person's voice as he or she is speaking. For example, pitch typically drops at the end of an utterance such as the one shown in Figures 8-11 through 8-13. The horizontal striations on the narrow-band spectrograms (Figures 8-11 and 8-13) become closer together at the end of the sentence, reflecting this drop in pitch. (As the pitch decreases, the harmonics come closer together.) If the utterance were a yes/no question instead, the striations would become farther apart as the pitch rose at the end of the sentence. In fact, this pitch rise can be seen on the word "dot," especially between about 700 and 850 ms, in Figure 8-14 (female asking "A tot, a dot?"). By the end of the question, we can see only one harmonic about every 500 Hz, indicating that the female's pitch has doubled from 250 to 500 Hz.

In certain clinical cases, the ability to measure changes in pitch can be very useful. Some people with autism, for example, exhibit sudden extreme pitch shifts. Figure 8-15 is a narrow-band spectrogram of a boy with autism pronouncing "badger" as [bæ- bæ- æ- æ- ædʒɚ]. Note the frequent breaks in his speech as well as the sharp rises in his harmonics. (The horizontal line at 900 Hz is simply a background hum.)

When we whisper, the vocal folds come close together, but they don't actually vibrate. When we have swollen or otherwise enlarged vocal cords (as with laryngitis, laryngeal warts, etc.), the vocal folds can't vibrate properly because they cannot meet smoothly. Either way, the glottal (source) wave doesn't have a well-defined spectrum (f_0 and harmonics), and therefore the amplifications of this spectrum will also be poorly defined, as illustrated in Figure 8-16. The vocal tract can only enhance the frequencies that it is given, so an imprecise glottal spectrum will yield imprecise formants. For this reason, spectrographs (and other acoustic analysis devices) are very valuable tools for diagnosing and treating voice disorders of various types. In the following chapter, we discuss spectrograms for different English speech sounds in more detail.

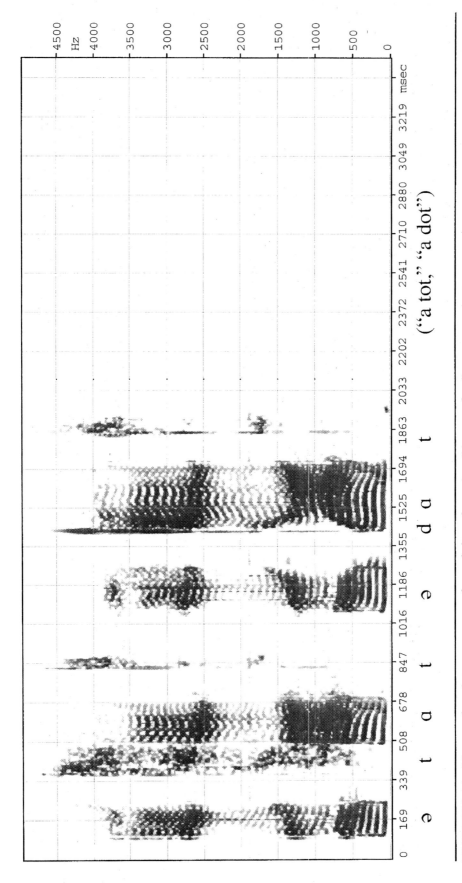

FIGURE 8-11 Narrow-band spectrogram of an adult male saying "A tot, a dot."

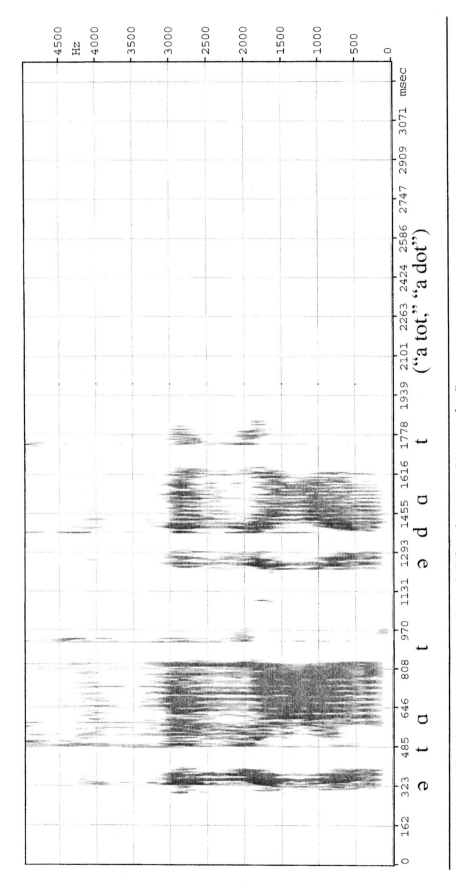

FIGURE 8-12 Wide-band spectrogram of an adult female saying "A tot, a dot."

109

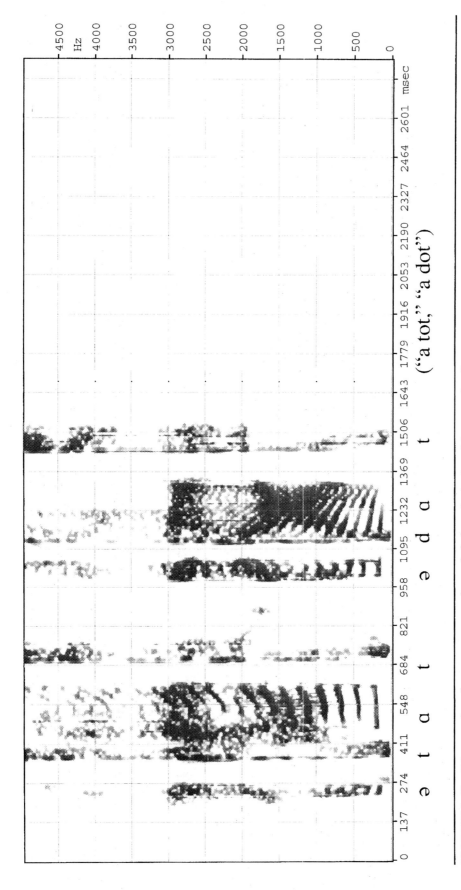

FIGURE 8-13 Narrow-band spectrogram of an adult female saying "A tot, a dot."

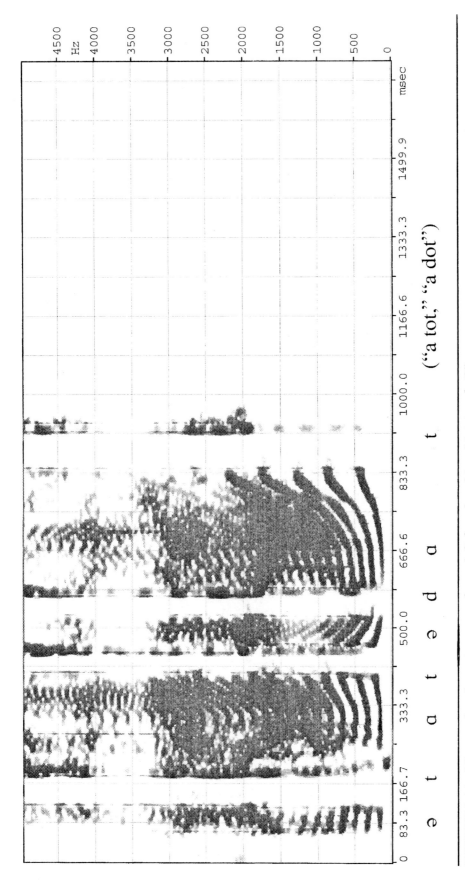

FIGURE 8-14 Narrow-band spectrogram of an adult female asking "A tot, a dot?"

111

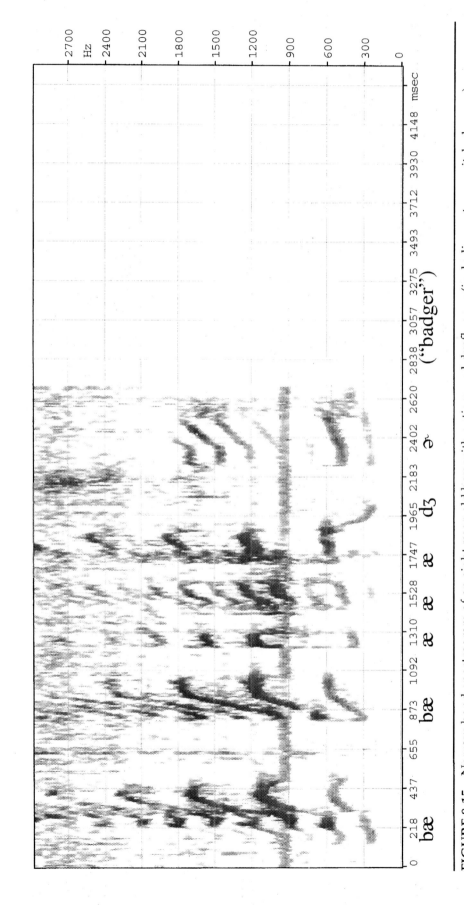

FIGURE 8-15 Narrow-band spectrogram of an eight-year-old boy with autism and dysfluency (including extreme pitch changes) producing the word "badger."

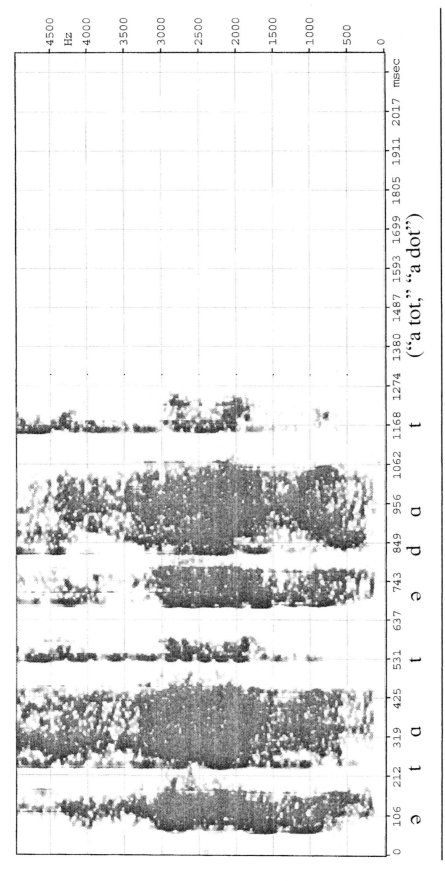

FIGURE 8-16 Narrow-band spectrogram of a hoarse adult female saying "A tot, a dot."

EXERCISES

1. The vocal tract includes

   a) lips.

   b) tongue.

   c) pharynx.

   d) lungs.

   e) all of the above.

   f) a, b, and c.

2. The Bernouilli effect causes

   a) the vocal folds to blow apart.

   b) the vocal folds to come together.

   c) the trachea to open.

   d) the pharyngeal air pressure to decrease.

   e) puffs of air to escape from the lungs.

3. People's pitches will rise if

   a) they exhale.

   b) their vocal folds are relaxed.

   c) their vocal folds are stretched.

   d) their vocal folds are swollen.

   e) their vocal folds are lengthened.

4. The frequency of a speaker's glottal pulses will influence

   a) the filter spectrum.

   b) the source spectrum.

   c) the output spectrum.

   d) a and c.

   e) b and c.

5. A lower f_0 will result in

   a) a denser source spectrum.

   b) a sparser (more spread out) source spectrum.

   c) a denser filter spectrum.

   d) a sparser filter spectrum.

   e) none of the above.

6. The resonant frequencies of a person's vocal tract will influence

   a) the filter spectrum.

   b) the source spectrum.

   c) the output spectrum.

   d) a and c.

   e) b and c.

7. On a spectrogram

    a) the vertical axis represents time.

    b) the horizontal axis represents amplitude.

    c) darkness represents frequency.

    d) all of the above.

    e) none of the above.

8. A wide-band spectrogram

    a) provides better frequency detail.

    b) provides better pitch detail.

    c) provides better time detail.

    d) provides better intensity detail.

    e) a and b.

9. Aperiodic sounds, as seen on a spectrogram,

    a) lack well-defined formants.

    b) are always very brief.

    c) are imperceptible.

    d) are most intense at very low frequencies.

    e) are only visible for voiced sounds.

Questions 10–12 refer to Figure 8-17, which shows the glottal wave of a person as a function of position at time $t = 0$ s. Assume that this wave can be constructed by Fourier's theorem using a harmonic series with all modes present. Assume that the speed of sound in air is 335m/s.

10. An observer is standing at the position $x = 20$ m listening to the glottal wave shown. What repeat time does the observer hear?

    a) 2/3 s

    b) 1/6 s

    c) 1/56 s

    d) 1/223 s

    e) none of these

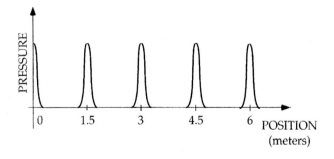

FIGURE 8-17   Glottal wave for Questions 10–12.

11. What is the repeat frequency of this glottal wave?

    a) 1.5 Hz

    b) 6 Hz

    c) 56 Hz

    d) 223 Hz

    e) none of the above

12. This is most likely the glottal wave of a

    a) woman.

    b) man.

    c) child.

    d) nonhuman.

For Questions 13–15, make two copies of Figure 8-18.

13. Suppose that a different glottal wave, still looking much like the one in Figure 8-17, but now of repeat frequency 200 Hz, is heard. Draw the source frequency spectrum of this new glottal wave using the envelope curve given in Figure 8-18. (Don't forget to label the frequencies on the horizontal axis.)

14. Suppose that this glottal wave is passed through a bandpass filter with a range of 350–820 Hz. Draw the resulting frequency spectrum of the filtered wave on your second copy of Figure 8-18. (Don't forget to label the frequencies on the horizontal axis.)

15. What is the repeat time of the filtered wave?

    Answer: _____ sec

Questions 16–17 refer to Figure 8-19, a pressure-time graph of a glottal wave.

16. Such a glottal wave of the voice determines

    a) the formants of a vowel sound.

    b) the quality of the speech sound.

    c) the pitch of the voice.

    d) the frequency of the unvoiced speech sounds.

    e) both b and c.

17. The speech sound associated with this glottal wave would have what repeat frequency?

    a) 0.007 Hz

    b) 70 Hz

    c) 125 Hz

    d) 143 Hz

    e) none of the above

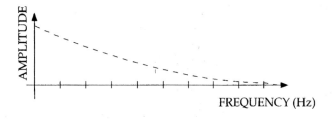

FIGURE 8-18 Envelope curve for Questions 13–14.

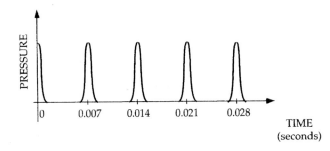

FIGURE 8-19   Pressure-time graph for Questions 16–17.

Questions 18–21 refer to the spectrograms in Figures 8-20 through 8-23. Fill in the blanks with the appropriate figure number.

18. The speaker in Figure _____ has the highest pitch.

19. The speaker in Figure _____ is asking a question.

20. The speaker in Figure _____ is probably either hoarse or whispering.

21. The speaker in Figure _____ is producing periodic sounds (vowels) only.

Questions 22–24 refer to the spectrogram in Figure 8-24.

22. This is a _____-band spectrogram.

23. An aperiodic sound can be identified near the area marked with the letter _____.

24. A decrease in pitch can be identified near the area marked with the letter _____.

For Questions 25–27, draw the figures on graph paper.

25. Draw the source (glottal wave) spectrum for a person with a fundamental frequency of 200 Hz.

26. Draw the resonance (filter) spectrum for a vocal tract that resonates at 200, 600, and 900 Hz.

27. Draw the output spectrum for the person in Question 25 speaking the vowel in Question 26.

28. On a narrow-band spectrogram of a vowel, 5 harmonics occur in the space of 1000 Hz. This person's fundamental frequency is
    a) 1000 Hz.
    b) 500 Hz.
    c) 10 Hz.
    d) 200 Hz.
    e) 5 Hz.

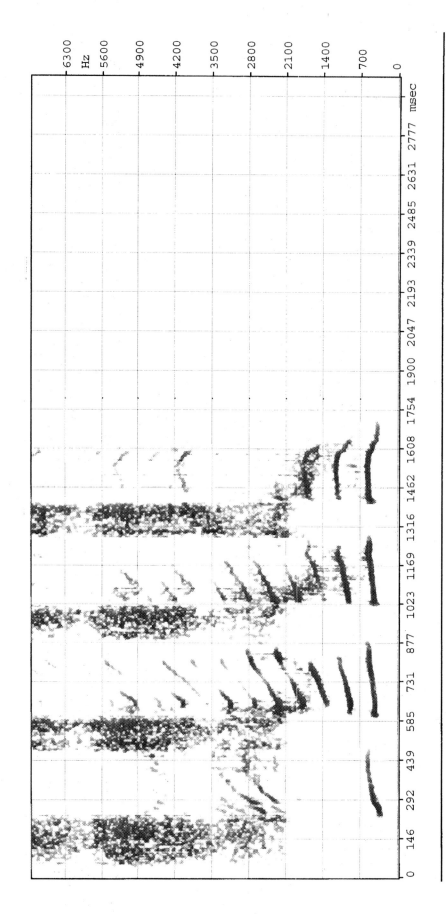

FIGURE 8-20 Spectrogram for Questions 18–21.

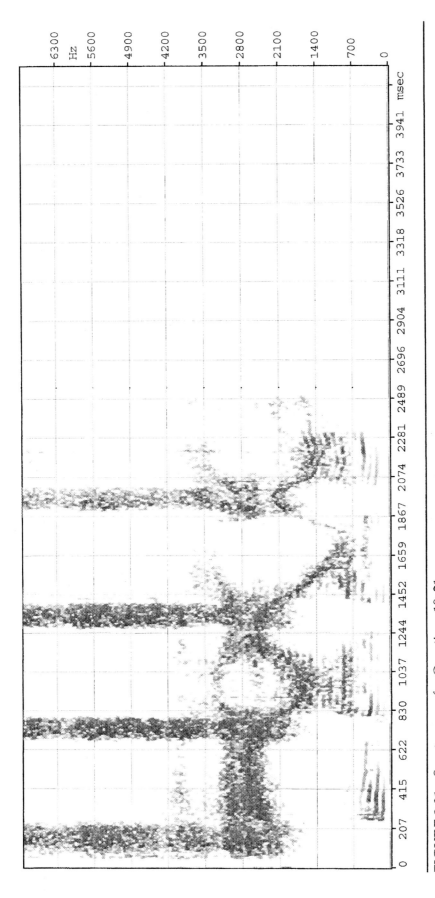

FIGURE 8-21 Spectrogram for Questions 18–21.

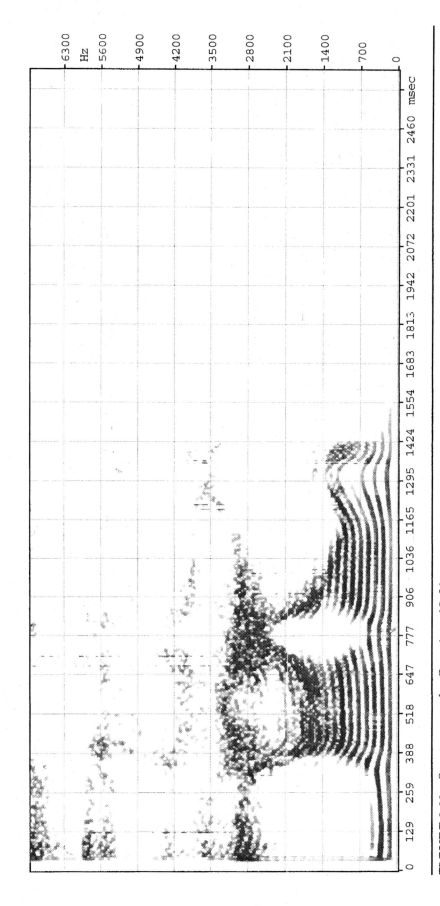

FIGURE 8-22 Spectrogram for Questions 18–21.

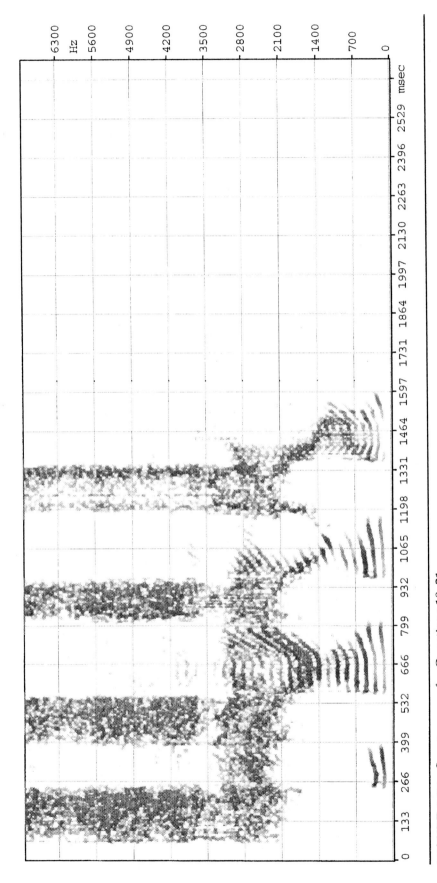

FIGURE 8-23 Spectrogram for Questions 18–21.

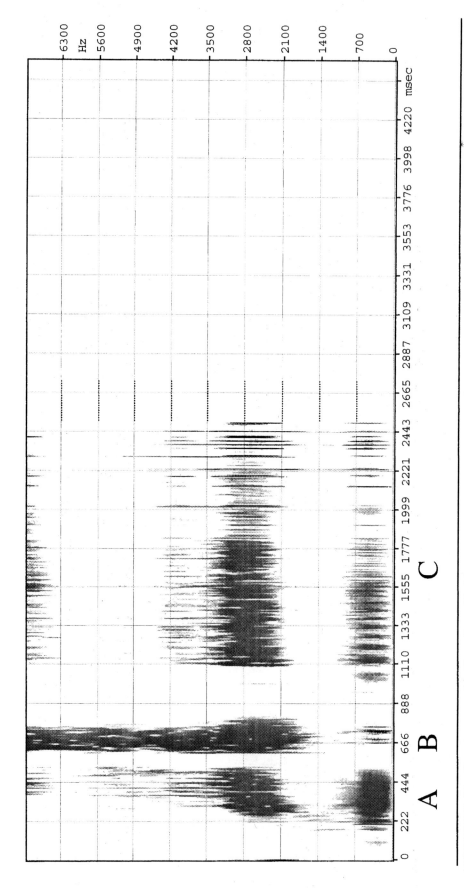

FIGURE 8-24 Spectrogram for Questions 22–24.

29. On a wide band spectrogram of a vowel, 10 glottal pulses occur in the space of 20 ms. This person's fundamental frequency is

    a) 1000 Hz.
    b) 500 Hz.
    c) 10 Hz.
    d) 200 Hz.
    e) 5 Hz.

Question 30 refers to the spectrograms in Figures 8-25 through 8-28.

30. Indicate which figure corresponds to each of the following song lines (as sung by an adult female).

    "My Bonnie lies over the ocean." _____
    "Fa la la la la la la la la." _____
    "I wanna hold your hand." _____
    "Mary had a little lamb." _____

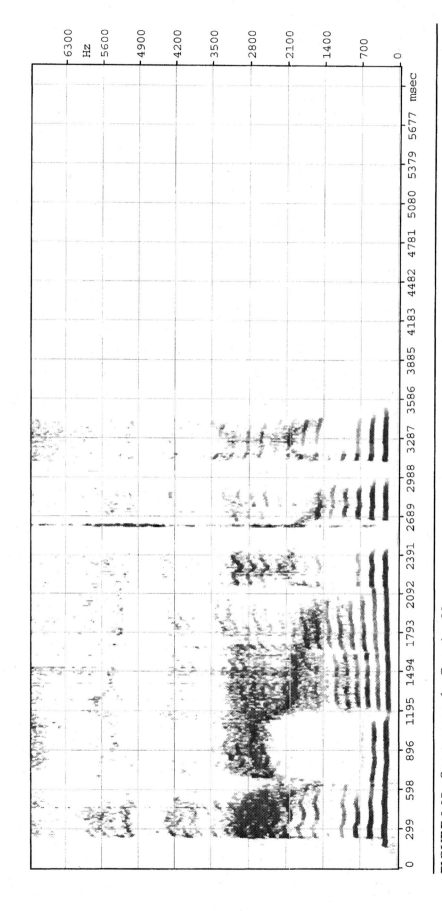

FIGURE 8-25 Spectrogram for Question 30.

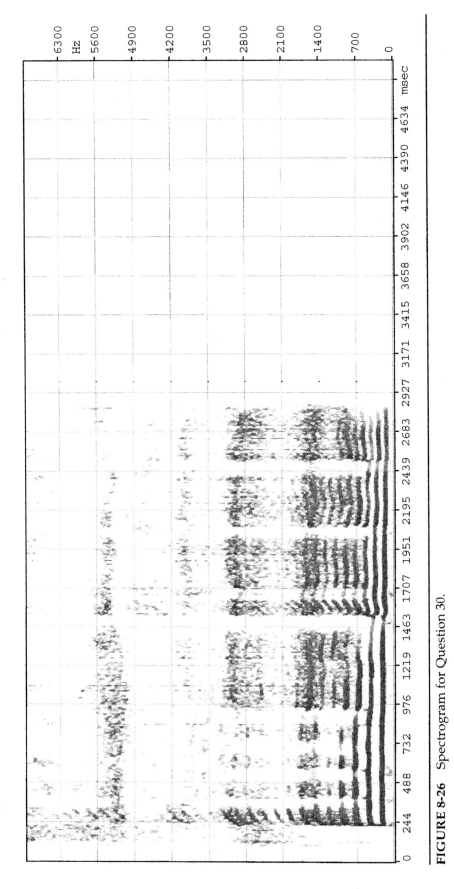

FIGURE 8-26 Spectrogram for Question 30.

125

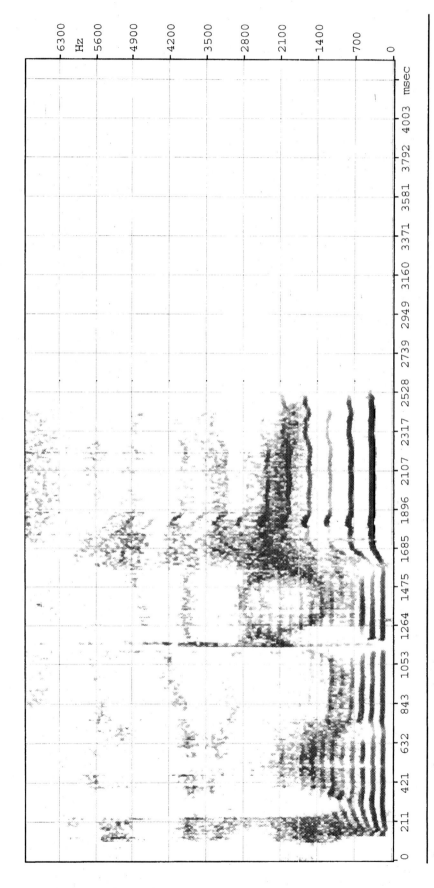

FIGURE 8-27 Spectrogram for Question 30.

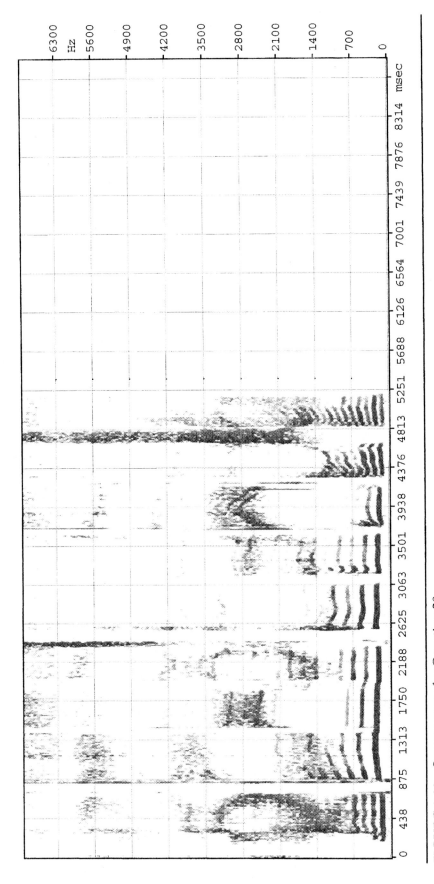

FIGURE 8-28 Spectrogram for Question 30.

127

9

Acoustics of Specific Speech Sounds

In this chapter we discuss how different speech sounds are made and their acoustic characteristics as seen on the spectrograms corresponding to those sounds.

9-A. Vowels

We have studied the properties of the vocal tract using vowels to model speech production. We have seen that they are the product of a glottal sound wave passing through a relatively open vocal tract. Vowels can be characterized into two types: pure vowels and diphthongs.

Pure vowels are those whose quality remains unchanged while we speak them, while diphthongs are vowel sounds whose quality changes, as the result of movements of the articulators, from the beginning to the end of articulation. The English pure vowels and diphthongs are shown in Table 9-1.

Figure 9-1 includes spectrograms of three pure vowel sounds—[i] ("ee"), [ɑ] ("ah"), and [u] ("ooh")—and Figure 9-2 shows a spectrogram of the diphthong [ɑɪ] (as in "eye"). Notice that the formants in the pure vowels remain relatively constant, and the formants in the diphthongs change frequencies over time as the diphthong is pronounced. The first two formants of the vowel [i] are spread widely apart, while the first two formants of the vowel [ɑ] are closer together. F_1 for [ɑ] is higher than for [i], and F_2 for [ɑ] is much lower than for [i]; sometimes the two formants seem to merge in the vowel [ɑ] because they are so close together. F_3 for [ɑ] is in the same frequency range as F_2 for [i]. The leftmost portion of the spectrogram for [ɑɪ] resembles that for [ɑ]; F_1 gradually falls, and F_2

TABLE 9-1 English Vowels and Diphthongs (in I.P.A.), with Examples

Pure Vowels	Diphthongs
i as in heed	eɪ as in hay
ɪ as in hid	oʊ as in hoe
ɛ as in head	ɑɪ as in high
æ as in had	ɑʊ as in how
ɑ as in hod	ɔɪ as in boy
ʊ as in hood	iɚ as in hear
u as in who	oɚ as in hoard
ʌ as in hub	ɑɚ as in hard
ə as in abide	eɚ as in hair
ɝ as in herb	uɚ as in tour
ɚ as in butter	

gradually rises until the formants are in position for [i].

The three "corner vowels," [ɑ], [i], [u], are the most distinctive pure vowels on a spectrogram. Diphthongs (especially [ɑɪ], [ɑʊ], [ɔɪ]—"eye," "ow," "oy") are also easy to identify as a group because of the extreme changes in their formants over time.

9-B. Consonants

Consonants are best described by specifying two features: place of articulation and manner of articulation. The places of articulation are the lips (**labial** consonants), the teeth (**dental** consonant), the ridge just be-

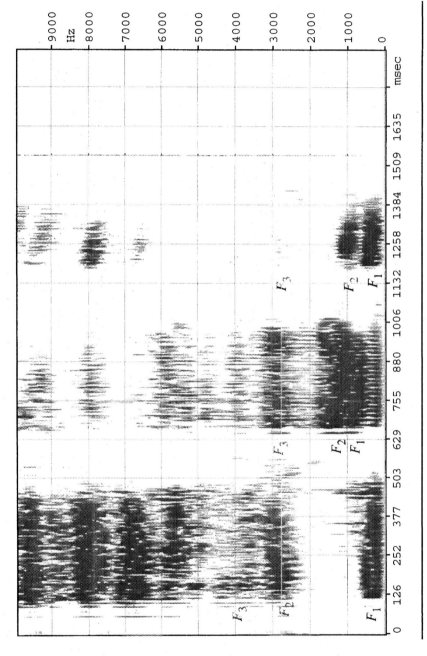

FIGURE 9-1 Wide-band spectrogram of an adult female saying [i], [ɑ], [u] ("ee," "ah," "ooh").

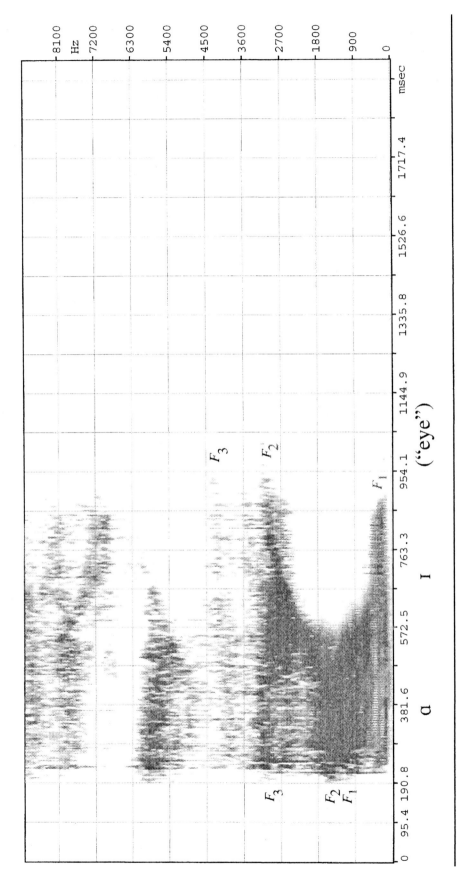

FIGURE 9-2 Wide-band spectrogram of an adult female saying [aɪ] ("eye").

TABLE 9-2   Classification of English Consonants in Terms of Place and Manner of Articulation

Place of Articulation	Manner of Articulation				
(Semivowel)	Plosive (Stop)	Fricative	Nasal	Liquid	Glide
Labial (lips only)	p, b (**pie, buy**)		m (**my**)		w (**why**)
Labio-Dental (teeth on lip)		f, v (**fie, vie**)			
Lingua-Dental (tongue tip between teeth)		θ, ð (**thigh, thy**)			
Alveolar (tongue tip on alveolar ridge)	t, d (**tie, die**)	s, z (**sigh, zoo**)	n (**nigh**)	l (**lie**)	j (**yes**)
Palatal (blade of tongue near hard palate)		ʃ, ʒ (**shy, measure**)		ɹ (**rye**)	
Velar (dorsum of tongue near velum)	k, g (**kite, guy**)		ŋ (**king**)		
Glottal (vocal folds brought close together)			h (**high**)		

Note: When two entries appear in the table, the left entry is unvoiced while the right entry is voiced.

hind the upper front teeth (**alveolar** consonants), the soft palate (**velar** consonants), and the glottis. The major categories of manner of articulation consist of **stops** (plosives), **fricatives**, **nasals**, **liquids**, and **glides** (semivowels). Table 9-2 classifies the different consonant sounds in terms of place and manner of articulation. Consonants are further distinguished by whether they are voiced or unvoiced. The acoustic features of each of these manners of articulation and their identification on spectrograms will be discussed in more detail below. We'll begin our discussion of the English consonant sounds with the glides and liquids, which are the most similar to vowels.

9-C. Glide and Liquid Consonants

The English glides (also called semivowels because of their very vowel-like nature)—[w] as in "why" and [j] as in "yes"—are produced by momentarily keeping the vocal tract in the position for articulating a vowel, and then rapidly changing it to the position of the following vowel in the syllable. Thus, glides must be followed by vowels. It is because of the smooth movement from one vowel to the next that they are called glides. The [j] glide is produced by initially shaping the vocal tract into a slight exaggeration of the position for the vowel [i] as in "heed," and the [w] glide is produced by initially shaping the vocal tract into a slight exaggeration of the position for the vowel [u] as in "hoot."

As seen in Figures 9-3 ([ji] [ju], "ye, you") and 9-4 ([wi] [wu], "we woo"), lighter but easily discernable formants can be identified during the glide portions

of the spectrograms of these syllables. Because the lips (for [w]) and tongue (for [j]) are only shaped and don't make close contact with other vocal structures, the vocal tract is still functioning as a (narrowed) tube, and therefore resonances (formants) are still visible. Because of the articulator movements that take place during the production of these sounds, significant changes are observed in their formant patterns on spectrograms. However, there is less change from the [j] to the [i] of [ji] than from the [j] to the [u] of [ju] because the tongue position for [j] is very similar to that of [i]. In a parallel fashion, there is less change from the [w] to the [u] of [wu] than from the [w] to the [i] of [wi] because the positions of the tongue and the lips for [w] are very similar to those for [u].

The liquid [l] is formed by putting the tip of the tongue against the gums and allowing air to pass to either side of the tongue (laterally), while at the same time vibrating the vocal folds. The resulting formant patterns (again, faint but still visible) are seen in Figure 9-5, in the syllables [li] [lu] ("lee, lou"). Note the strong first formants and weak second formants of the [l]s. The F_2 becomes stronger and quickly rises for the [i] vowel (which, as we saw above, has a very high F_2), and becomes stronger with a very gradual fall for the [u] vowel (which has a lower F_2).

The [ɹ] sound in American English is articulated in two possible ways: either by bunching the back of the tongue up towards the soft palate, or by curling the tongue tip back. Both positions yield the same sound. The formants for [ɹ] are fairly strong, with a low F_3, as is especially visible in the leftmost word of Figure 9-6, "ree."

A common speech difficulty in English speakers

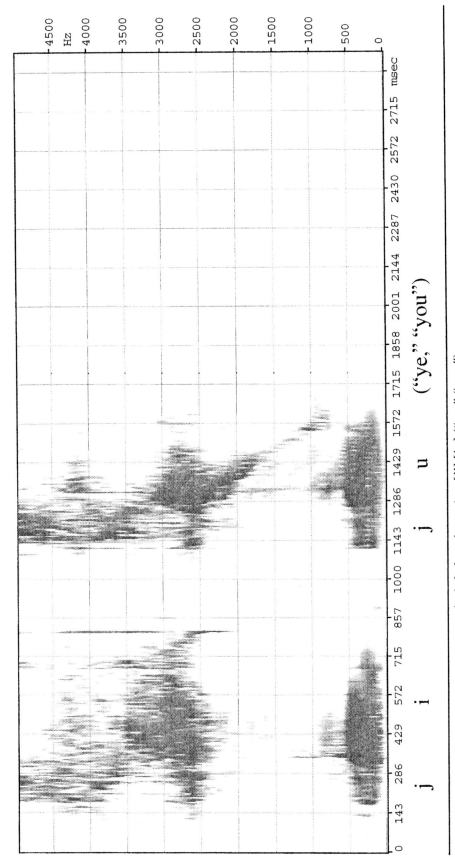

FIGURE 9-3 Wide-band spectrogram of adult female saying [ji] [ju] ("ye," "you").

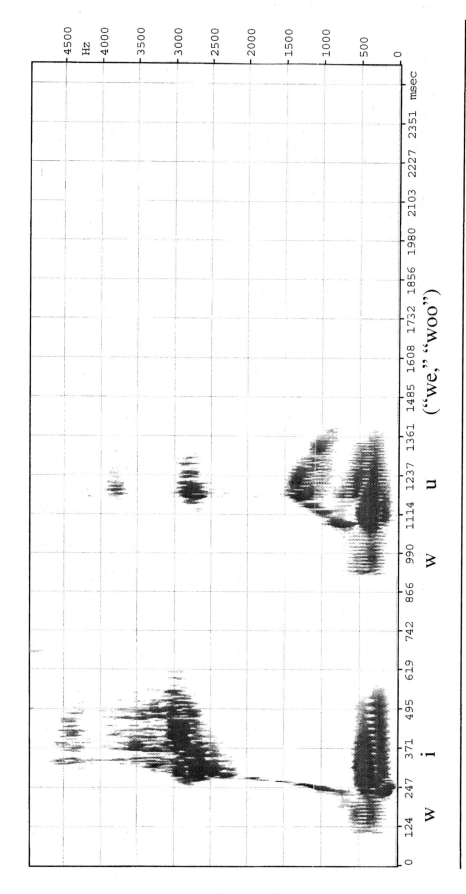

FIGURE 9-4 Wide-band spectrogram of adult female saying [wi] [wu] ("we" "woo").

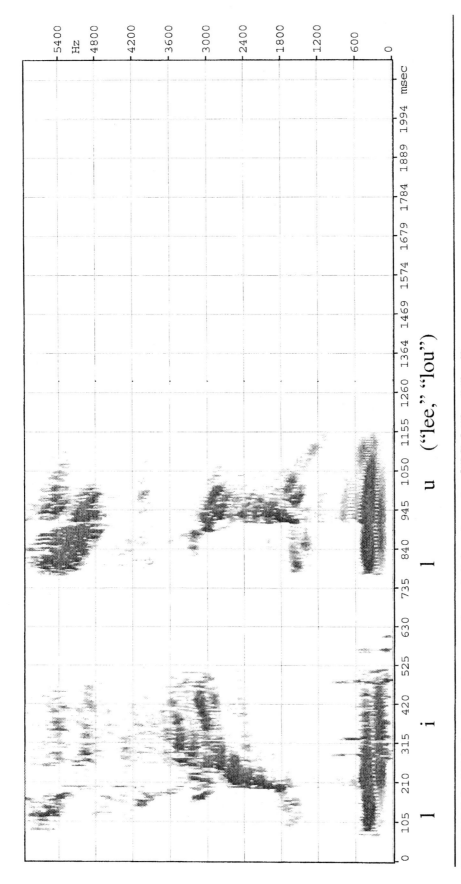

FIGURE 9-5 Wide-band spectrogram of an adult female saying [li] [lu] ("lee," "lou").

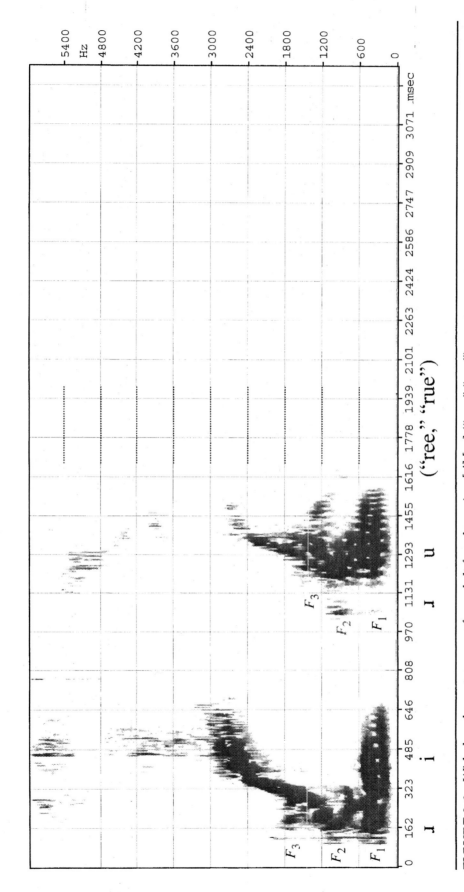

FIGURE 9-6 Wide-band spectrogram of an adult female saying [ɹi] [ɹu] ("ree," "rue").

is the immature production of the consonant /ɹ/. To the untrained ear, an immature /ɹ/ sounds very like [w]. However, acoustic studies have shown that children who misarticulate /ɹ/ often produce a sound that is actually acoustically in between [ɹ] and [w], transcribed [ɹ]. Figure 9-7 illustrates these three sounds, in the words [ɹɪ ŋ], [ɹɪ ŋ], and [w ɪ ŋ] ("ring", "ring" with immature [ɹ] sound, "wing"). Note that the formants for [w] are the weakest, indicating that this speaker produces [w] with more constriction than [ɹ].

9-D. *Nasal Consonants*

The nasal consonants are articulated by lowering the soft palate, thereby connecting the nasal cavity to the pharynx, and by blocking the mouth at the lips or with the tongue. Because the air is prevented from going through the oral cavity, these sounds are sometimes referred to as nasal stops. However, the air is able to flow freely through the nasal cavity, so (faint) formants can often be seen. As a result of the closure of the oral cavity, the vocal tract for nasals runs from the larynx to the nostrils instead of from the larynx to the lips. This is a longer tube, which therefore resonates at lower frequencies. In addition, much more damping goes on in the nasal cavities because of the soft and uneven material therein. Thus, one result of opening the nasal cavity is to significantly decrease the intensity of the formants, especially in the 800–2000 Hz range, which is the frequency range of the second formant for most vowels. Another result is lower resonant frequencies—that is, lower formants in general because of the increased length of the vocal tract. Therefore, there are two signatures of a nasal consonant or a nasalized vowel. The first signature is that the intensity of the formants, especially the second formant, becomes very low during the nasal stretch; the second is that the frequency of the first formant comes down during the nasal stretch.

Since the nostrils are not as efficient as the mouth in projecting sound energy, the overall intensity level of the nasal consonants is lowered even more. This means that the formants of nasal consonants will be lighter, usually much lighter, in color than the vowel formants. The spectrogram in Figure 9-8 of the syllables [lɑ], [nɑ] ("la, na") illustrates the difference in intensity of a nasal consonant in comparison to a liquid, especially at the level of F_2. Notice from the presence of (very faint) striations that all nasals are voiced consonants.

A clinical voice problem that is often encountered by speech-language pathologists is the production of speech with excessive nasality. This is most clearly exemplified in persons with cleft palate, as there is an opening from their oral cavities into their nasal cavities. Therefore, air always passes through both cavities, giving a nasal resonance to all speech sounds. Again, speech-language pathologists often use acoustic analysis to verify their subjective impressions of nasality. Figure 9-9 shows two productions of "a tot," first with excess nasality ([ə̃ tã t]), and then spoken normally.

Although many Americans refer to people who have colds as speaking nasally, a blocked nasal cavity actually prevents air from escaping by that route, even when it should (i.e., for nasal consonants). Therefore, most people with colds actually speak in a **denasal** fashion, with nasal consonants that have less nasal resonance than they normally would (e.g., the word "mom" sounds more like "Bob") because the air is blocked from passing through the nasal passages. The spectrogram in Figure 9-10 illustrates this similarity; the spectrogram of "mom" with a stuffy nose looks much more like "Bob" than like "mom" with a clear nose.

9-E. *Fricative Consonants*

The fricative consonants are made by constricting the air flow in the mouth so as to make the air turbulent. This results in a hissing sound. The constriction of the air for a fricative is enough that resonance cannot occur during the production of these consonants. Therefore, formants are not seen.

Each fricative place of articulation involves a different type of constriction. For example, the labiodental fricative [f] in "fie" is articulated by forming a constriction between the upper teeth and the lower lip; the lingua-dental fricative [θ] in "thigh" has a constriction between the tip of the tongue and teeth; the alveolar [s] in "sigh" is the result of a constriction between the tongue tip and the alveolar ridge; and the palatal [ʃ] in "shy" is articulated by forming a constriction between the blade of the tongue and the hard palate. The glottal fricative "h" is articulated by expelling air through the mostly open glottis and vocal tract. These are the voiceless fricatives.

Although the fricatives as a group are usually easy to distinguish in spectrograms due to their relatively long vertical bands of high-frequency energy, distinguishing one fricative from another is not as

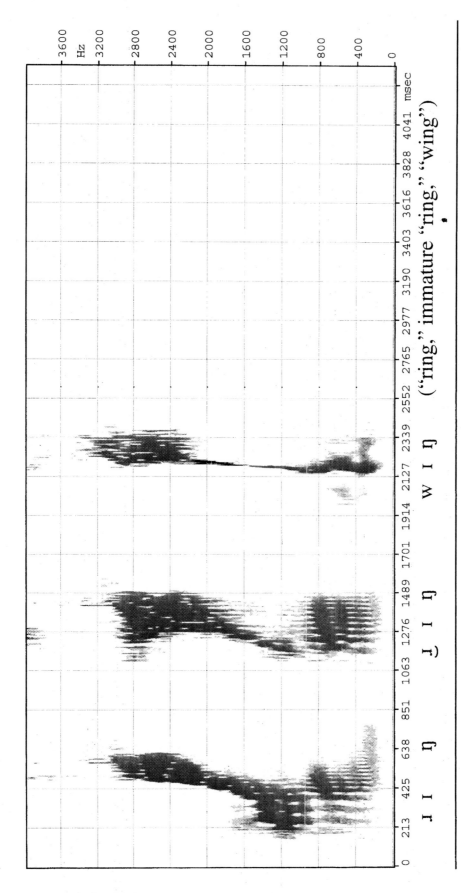

FIGURE 9-7 Wide-band spectrogram of an adult female saying [ɹɪŋ], [ɹɪŋ], [wɪŋ] ("ring" normally and with immature production, "wing").

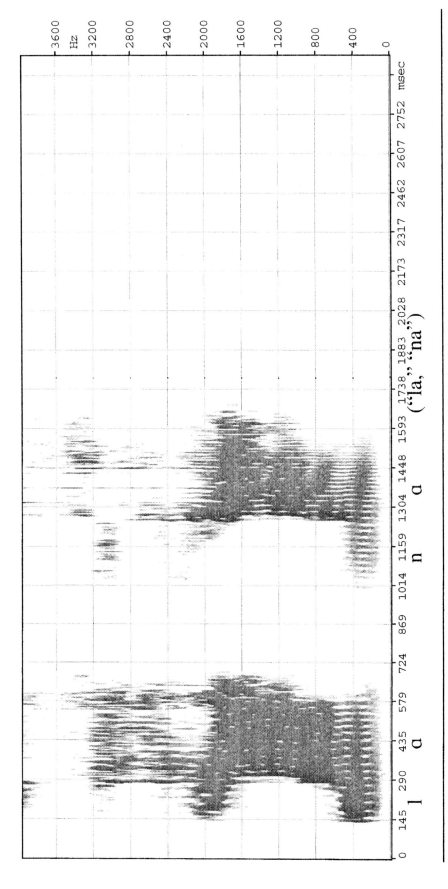

FIGURE 9-8 Wide-band spectrogram of an adult female saying [lɑ], [nɑ] ("la," "na").

139

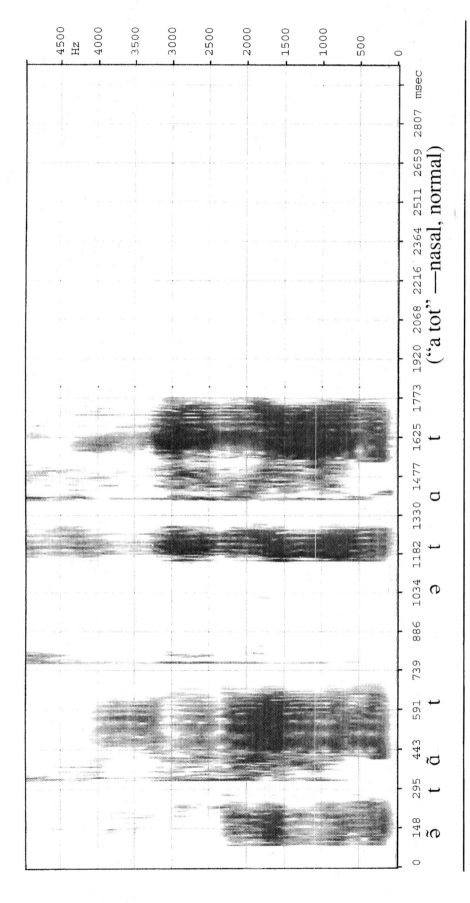

FIGURE 9-9 Wide-band spectrogram of an adult female saying [ɑ̃ tɑ̃t], [ə tɑt] ("a tot" with excess nasality, then normally).

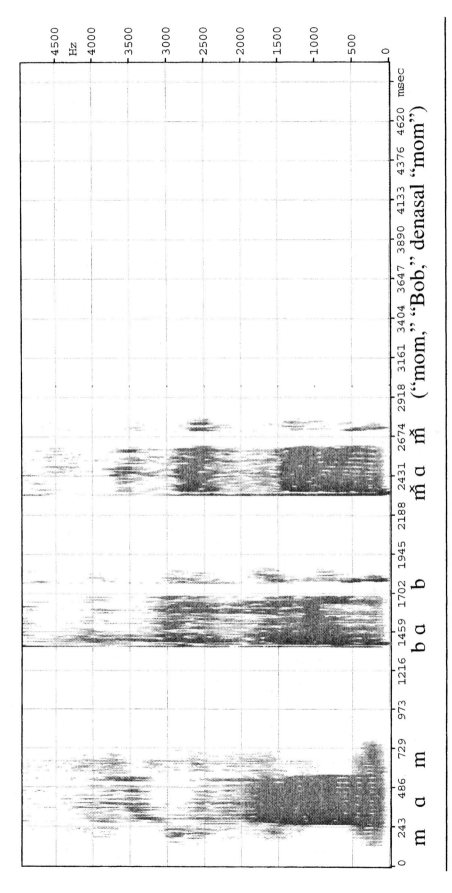

FIGURE 9-10 Spectrogram of "mom," "Bob," and denasal "mom."

easy. The exact range of the noise bands they create is one way to do so. For the palatal fricative [ʃ] as produced by a female speaker, for example, the frequency of the noise band ranges from 2000 to 8000 Hz, as shown in Figure 9-11. For [s] the frequencies below about 4500 Hz are filtered out, but the band extends upwards beyond 10,000 Hz. Both [f] and [θ] have most of their noise energy in the high-frequency range of 8000 Hz and above (beyond the top of the spectrogram). The glottal fricative [h] has very low-frequency noise, between 1000 and 2000 Hz. The reason for these differences is that the location of the constriction in the vocal tract tube determines the frequency of the hissing noise that results. In all cases, the noise spreads over a range of frequencies, but the farther front the constriction, the higher the frequency range. If we consider our tube model, this makes sense. The fricative noise created at the glottis for [h] travels through a long tube before reaching the outside air, and is therefore low-frequency. The farther front the constriction, the shorter the tube that the fricative noise will pass through, and the higher its frequency. Thus, as shown in Figure 9-11, the noise frequency decreases as the speaker progresses from the most front fricative [f] (for which there is essentially no tube at all) to the most back fricative [h].

Another distinction among the fricatives is the intensity of the noise associated with different types of fricatives. The hissing of the dental fricatives ([f] and [θ]) results from squeezing the air through a wide, flat opening (either the top teeth on the bottom lip or the tongue between the teeth), and therefore they are quiet. For [h], the air is passing through a fairly open glottis, so its noise is generally even quieter. Sometimes these fricatives are barely visible on a spectrogram. The hissing of the **sibilant** fricatives [s] and [ʃ] is due to the air's being forced through a very narrow channel (a groove created by the tongue) as well as past a straight, hard obstacle (the teeth), resulting in a much louder sound. These differences in noise intensity can be seen in Figure 9-11.

The production of the [s] sound requires a great deal of precision in English because the speaker has to ensure that the listener hears [s], not [ʃ] or [θ]. (Few languages have as many voiceless fricatives as English, probably for this reason.) Therefore, a lisp can be a significant speech problem for an English speaker. There are two types of lisps that speech-language pathologists treat: a frontal lisp ([s̪]—the "all I want for Christmas is my two front teeth" sound) and a lat-

eral lisp, which is produced with the tongue too flat (as if for the production of [l]) against the alveolar ridge, yielding a very wet sound [ɬ]). As shown in Figure 9-12, these misarticulations of the /s/ alter the acoustic properties of the fricative noise. The noise band for a fronted /s/ is higher (because the tube in front of the constriction is shorter) and weaker, more like [θ]. The noise band for a lateralized /s/ is lower, and some high-frequency formants are visible, more like a cross between [ʃ] and [l].

Of course, these are not the only fricative sounds in our language. English has an almost-complete set of voiced fricatives, as well. Before we can discuss these, we take a detour through the differences between voiced and voiceless consonants: **Voiced** describes speech sounds during which the vocal folds are vibrating. The vocal folds are not continuously vibrating during speech production; in fact, they vibrate only about 70 percent of the time. When we whisper, they are vibrating very little or not at all. Certain consonants are always **voiceless** (or **unvoiced**), whether they are whispered or not, which means that the vocal folds are simply open during their production. Thus, a voiced consonant is one articulated with the vocal folds vibrating, whereas a voiceless consonant is one articulated without vibrating the vocal folds. The primary signature of a voiced sound in a spectrogram is the presence of the **voice bar**—a dark band of energy at the very bottom of the spectrogram, reflecting the fundamental frequency of the person's voice. The voiced fricatives are [v] as in "vie," [ð] as in "thy," [z] as in "zoo," and [ʒ] as in "measure." (The voiced palatal fricative [ʒ] does not occur at the beginnings of English words; English lacks a voiced glottal fricative phoneme.) When we compare the spectrogram of "fee, thee [with voiceless "th"], see, she, he" in Figure 9-11 to that of "vee, thee [with voiced "th"], zee, zhee" in Figure 9-13, we can see these voice bars below the consonantal noise components of the syllables (weakest for "zee" as produced by this speaker). In other respects, the noise bands for voiced fricatives are very similar to those for voiceless fricatives (though they do tend to be a little bit less intense).

9-F. *Stop Consonants*

The plosive consonants, otherwise known as the stop consonants, are made by blocking the air pressure in the vocal tract and then suddenly releasing it.

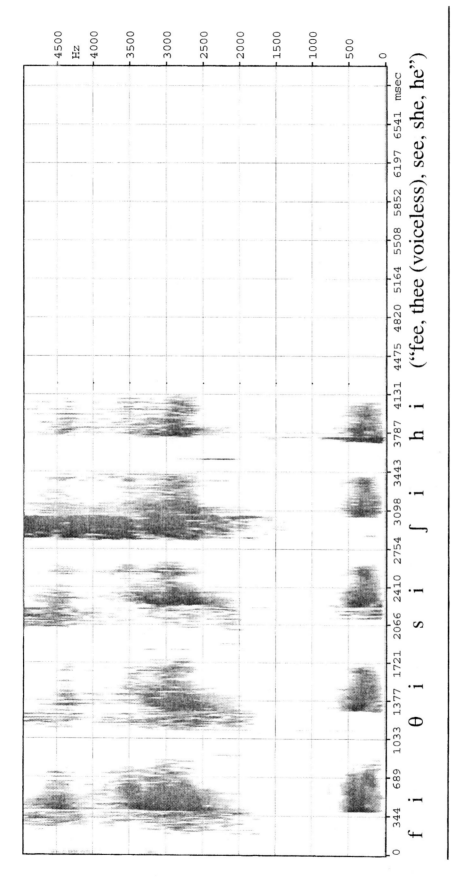

FIGURE 9-11 Wide-band spectrogram of an adult female saying [fi], [θi], [si], [ʃi], [hi] ("fee," "thee" [with a voiceless "th" sound], "see," "she," "he").

143

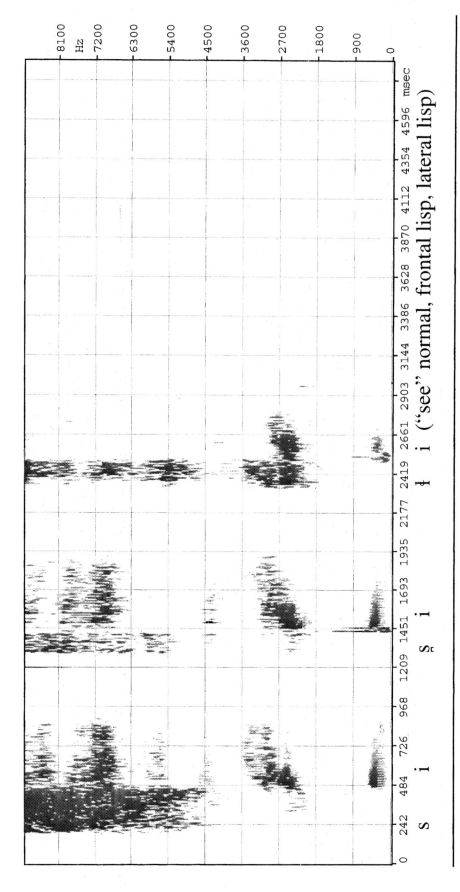

FIGURE 9-12 Wide-band spectrogram of an adult female saying [si], [s̪i], [l̪i] ("see" normally, with a frontal lisp, with a lateral lisp).

144

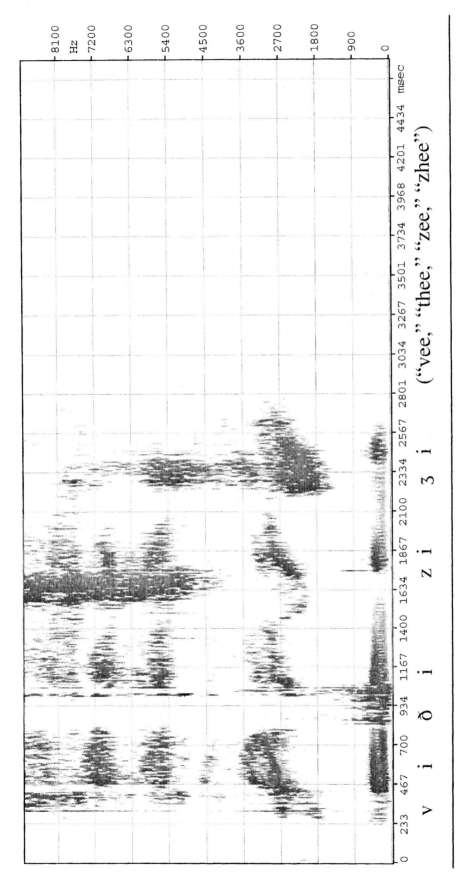

FIGURE 9-13 Wide-band spectrogram of an adult female saying [vi], [ði], [zi], [ʒi] ("vee," "thee" [with voiced "th"], "zee," "zhee").

145

Therefore, a stop is characterized by a short silence, or near silence, followed by a short burst of noise. As with the fricatives, stops occur in voiceless-voiced pairs. There are three voiced plosives [b, d and g], and three voiceless plosives [p, t, and k]. Both include a short period of silence during the closure, but they differ in the length of that silent period. We perceive the voiced stops to be voiced because the voicing begins earlier than for the voiceless stops; the silence is shorter, and therefore we have less opportunity to hear the (voiceless) burst of air that occurs when the consonant is released. Instead, we hear the beginning of the vowel because the voicing has begun. Thus, the silent stage of a plosive lasts between 0.07 and 0.14 seconds, with the shorter silences corresponding to the voiced plosives. The time between the release of the air (the burst) and the beginning of voicing is called the **voice onset time** of the consonant. Voice onset time varies from one place of articulation to another and from one language to another, but voiced consonants always have a shorter voice onset time than voiceless consonants in the same language.

Once the voicing begins, the silence ends. During the burst, the noise energy is spread widely over the spectrum, but the distribution of energy tends to occur at different frequency regions according to the place of articulation of the consonant. In the labial [p] and [b] consonants, for example, the sound intensity is concentrated in the low-frequency range (600–800 Hz). The sound intensity for the velar [k] and [g] consonants peaks near the middle frequencies (1800–2000 Hz), and the sound intensity for the alveolar [t] and [d] consonants peaks at high frequencies (near 4000 Hz). The sound intensity is higher for the voiced plosives than for the unvoiced plosives. The spectrograms in Figures 9-14 and 9-15 illustrate the voiceless and voiced stop consonants respectively in the syllables [pi] [ti] [ki] ("pea," "tea," "key") and [bi] [di] [gi] ("bee," "dee," "ghee"). Note the differences in the frequencies of the noise bands (lowest for the labials, highest for the alveolars) and that the noise bands are darker (louder) for the voiceless stops. Note also that the voicing in the "b," "d," and "g" shows up as initial low-frequency sounds before or around the same time as the vertical band that reflects the burst of energy when the consonant sound is released. In addition, striations are visible across the transition from the burst to the vowel in these voiced consonants. The unvoiced sounds simply have initial silence before and after the noise burst because the vocal folds are not vibrating.

9G. Coarticulation

Although many of the spectrograms you will see will break up the horizontal time axis into regions corresponding to particular sounds, it is important to keep in mind that this is only meant as a general guide. It is incorrect to pick off a particular time gap in the spectrogram and say this is such-and-such a vowel or consonant because, when we speak, sounds get blended together and it would be inaccurate to say that a certain sound started at some particular time and ended at some other particular time. For example, the sounds in the word "warrior" shown in Figure 9-16 overlap so much that it would be very difficult to say where each one begins (except the [w]) or ends (except the final [ɚ]).

In addition, we speak very rapidly, so we don't have time to carefully enunciate every consonant and vowel in a word. It takes time to transition from one articulatory position to another, so one speech sound in a word may be affected by the preceding or (more commonly in English) the following sound. For example, the [s] fricative noise in "see" is slightly higher than that in "Sue" because the upcoming vowel F_2 is lower in "Sue," as seen in Figure 9-17. Our lips begin to round (lengthening the tube in front of the [s] constriction) before we are finished producing the [s] sound. Similarly, the frequency of the noise burst for [t] in "twin" is lower than the frequency for the [t] in "tin," as Figure 9-18 illustrates. Acoustically, this makes sense because the second formant for [ɪ] is much higher than that for [w]. Articulatorily, this makes sense because once again the lips begin to get ready for the [w] (thereby lengthening the tube in front of the [t] constriction) before the [t] sound is complete. Stop bursts can also be affected by the following vowel. For example, the burst for [p] is higher before [i] (which has a higher F_2) than before [u]. Similarly, the burst for [k] is lower for [u] (which has a lower F_2) than before [i]. As a result, as can be seen in Figure 9-19, the bursts for [p] before [i] and [k] before [u] end up in a similar frequency range.

The velum (soft palate) moves particularly slowly relative to the other articulators. In English, we typically start to lower the velum (to close off the oral cavity and open the nasal cavity) in advance of a nasal consonant. Therefore, vowels that occur before nasal consonants tend to be nasalized, with some of the associated features of nasalization: decreased amplitude (especially for F_2) and lower formants. This is evident when the vowel portions of "man" and "pat" are compared in Figure 9-20.

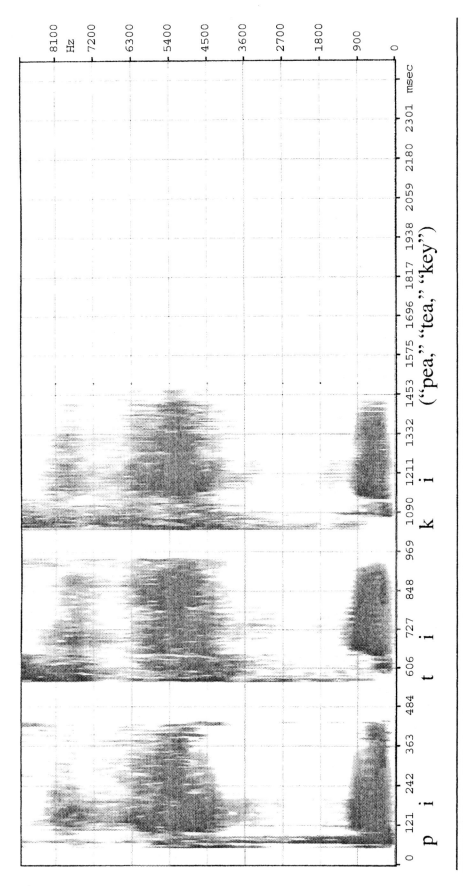

FIGURE 9-14 Wide-band spectrogram of an adult female saying [pi] [ti] [ki] ("pea," "tea," "key").

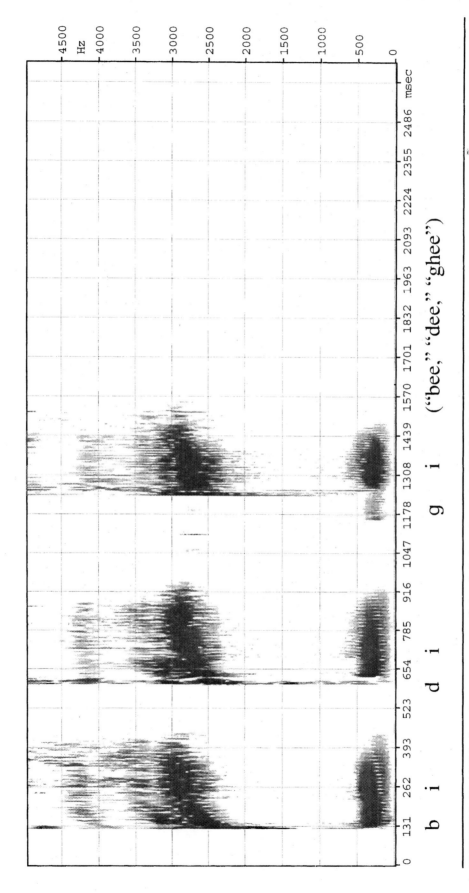

FIGURE 9-15 Wide-band spectrogram of an adult female saying [bi] [di] [gi] ("bee," "dee," "ghee").

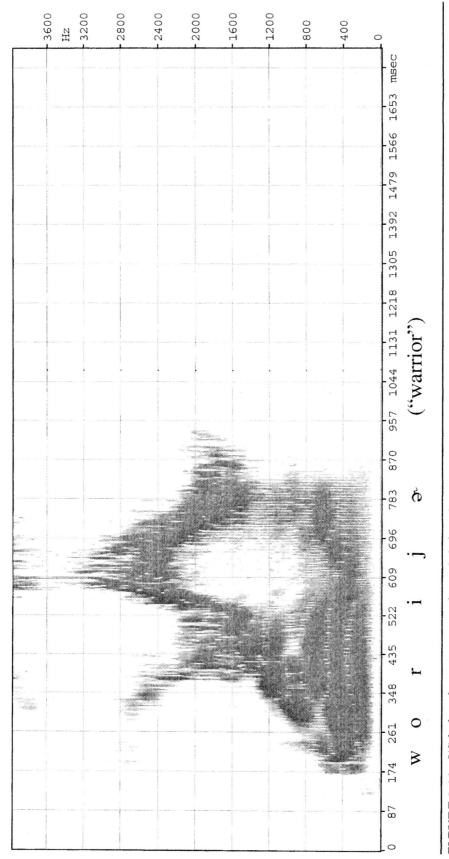

FIGURE 9-16 Wide-band spectrogram of an adult female saying "warrior."

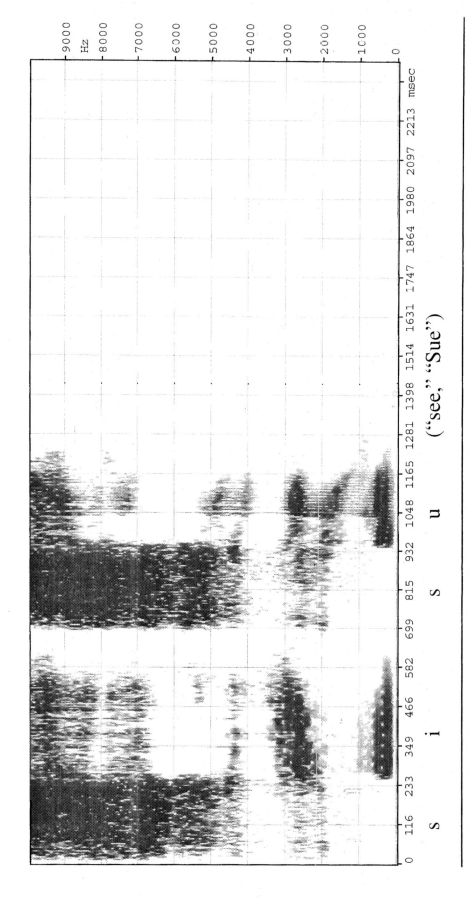

FIGURE 9-17 Wide-band spectrogram of an adult female saying [si] [su] ("see," "Sue").

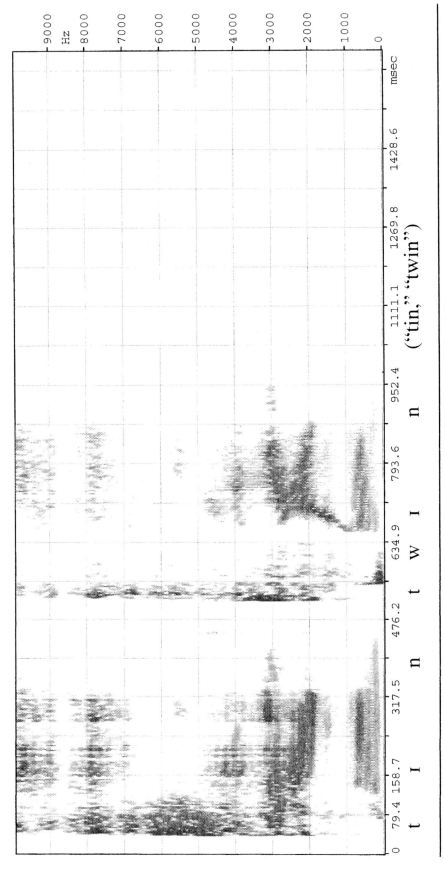

FIGURE 9-18 Wide-band spectrogram of an adult female saying [tɪn] [twɪn] ("tin," "twin")

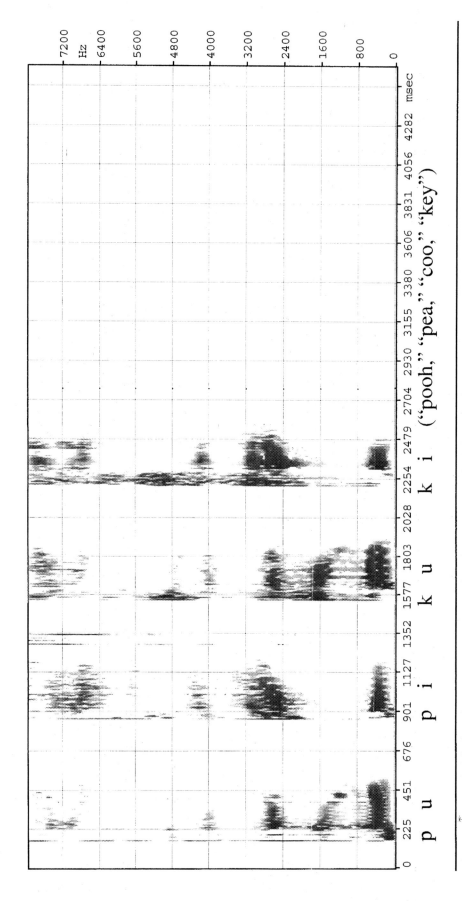

FIGURE 9-19 Wide-band spectrogram of an adult female saying [pu] [pi] [ku] [ki] ("pooh," "pea," "coo," "key").

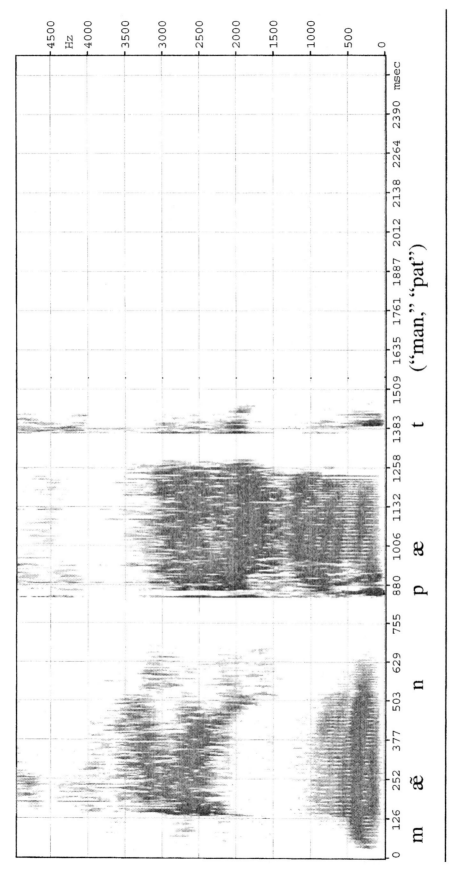

FIGURE 9-20 Wide-band spectrogram of an adult female saying [mæ̃n] [pæt] ("man," "pat").

EXERCISES

1. Consider the spectrograms in Figure 9-21. Fill in the blanks with the letters (A, B, C, D) from the spectrogram to indicate which word matches each description.

   _____ contains a diphthong

   _____ and _____ begin with a voiceless stop

   _____ ends with a nasal

   _____ shows the word [to] ("toe")

   _____ shows the word [ki] ("key")

   _____ shows the word [dʌm] ("dumb")

   _____ shows the word [gɑɪ] ("guy")

2. In French, the nasalization of the vowel can change the meaning of the word. For example, the words "beau" ([bo]) and "bon" ([bõ)]) are identical, except that the vowel in "bon" is nasalized (the "n" at the end of "bon" is not pronounced). Which of the words in Figure 9-22 is "bon" (A or B)?

3. Indicate the figure number that corresponds with each of the following sentences.

   Set A: (Figures 9-23, 9-24, 9-25, 9-26, and 9-27)

   Sound Scope channel A. _____

   The "d" is on the "t." _____

   You went where? _____

   He and she see the fee. _____

   Sue threw loose noodles on cue. _____

   Set B: (Figures 9-28, 9-29, 9-30, 9-31, 9-32)

   Mom shops for pots of cod. _____

   Can you come? _____

   Channel B Sound Scope. _____

   We were away a year ago. _____

   I don't want to sew it up. _____

4. A high F_2 is a good cue for which sound?

   a) [t]

   b) [i]

   c) [θ]

   d) [ɑ]

   e) [m]

5. In a spectrogram of the sound _____, distinct first and second formants always can be seen.

   a) [t]

   b) [i]

   c) [θ]

   d) [ɑ]

   e) [m]

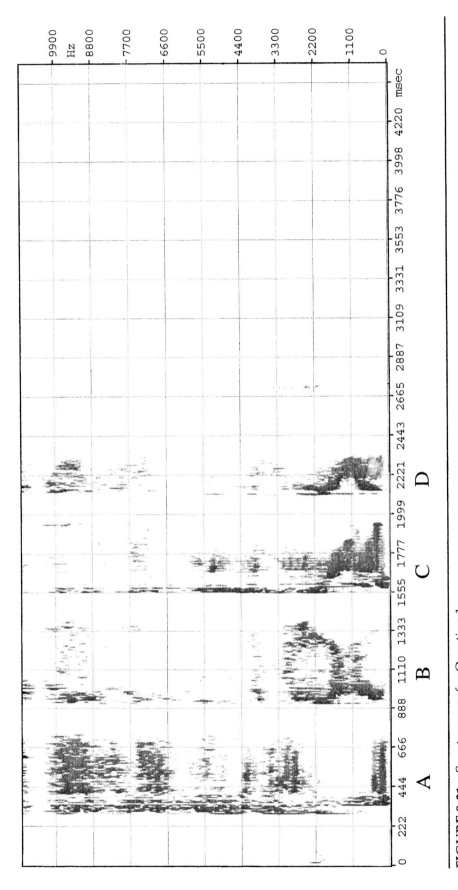

FIGURE 9-21 Spectrogram for Question 1.

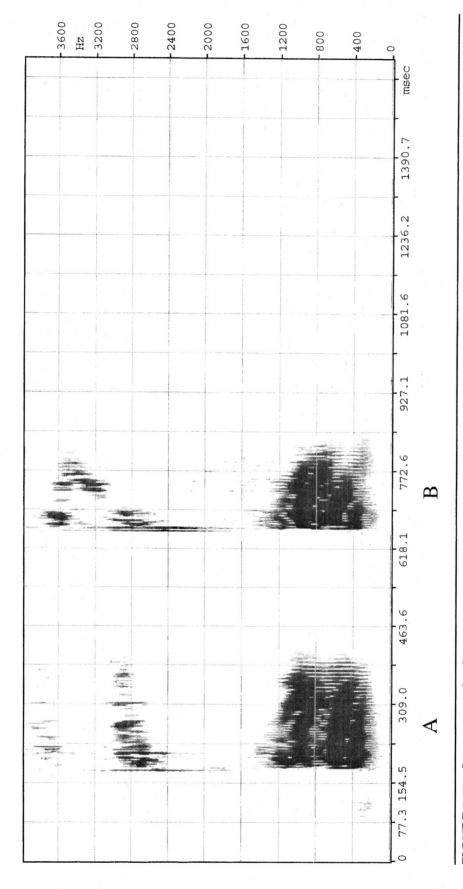

FIGURE 9-22 Spectrogram for Question 2.

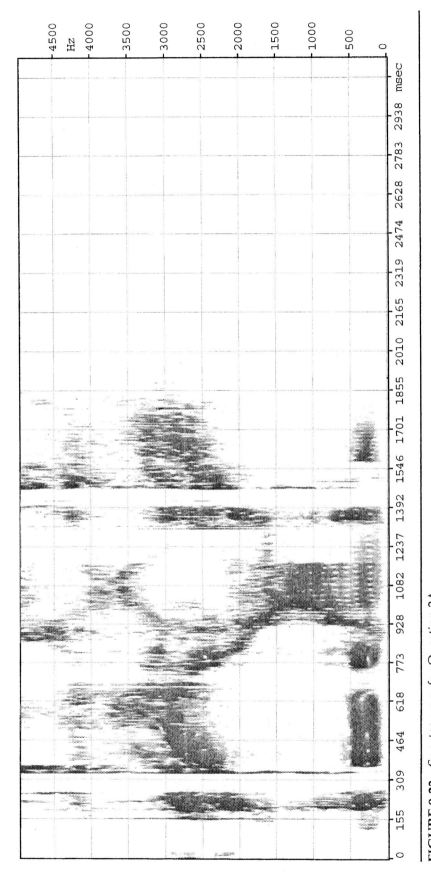

FIGURE 9-23 Spectrogram for Question 3A.

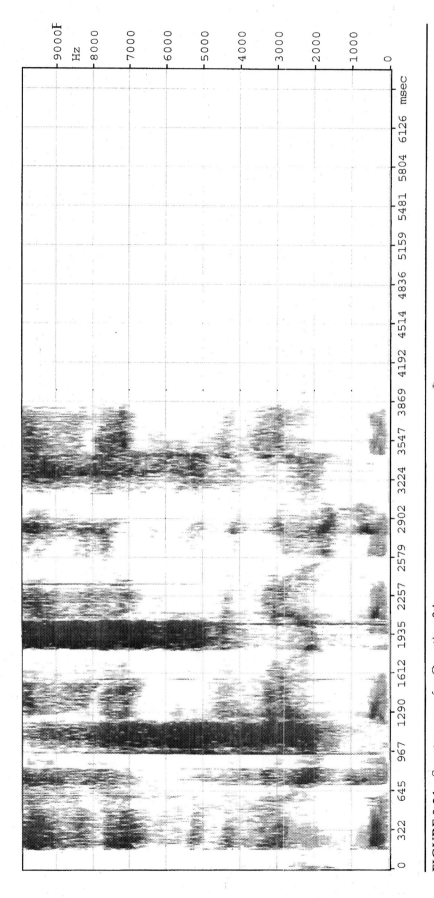

FIGURE 9-24 Spectrogram for Question 3A.

158

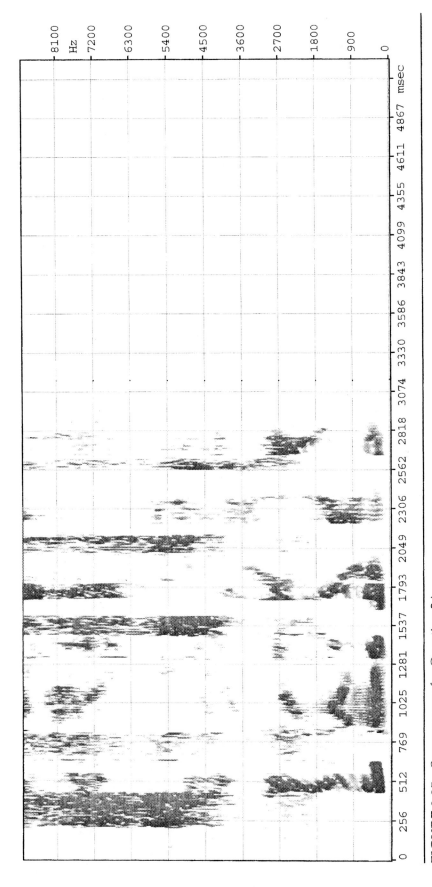

FIGURE 9-25 Spectrogram for Question 3A.

159

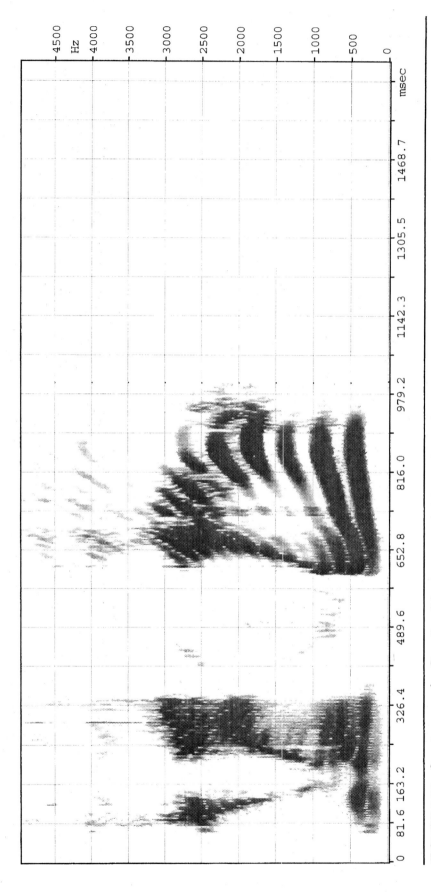

FIGURE 9-26 Spectrogram for Question 3A.

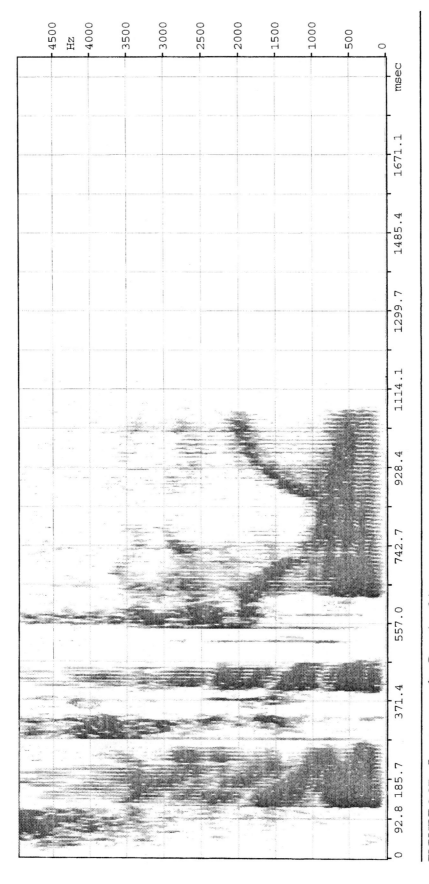

FIGURE 9-27 Spectrogram for Question 3A.

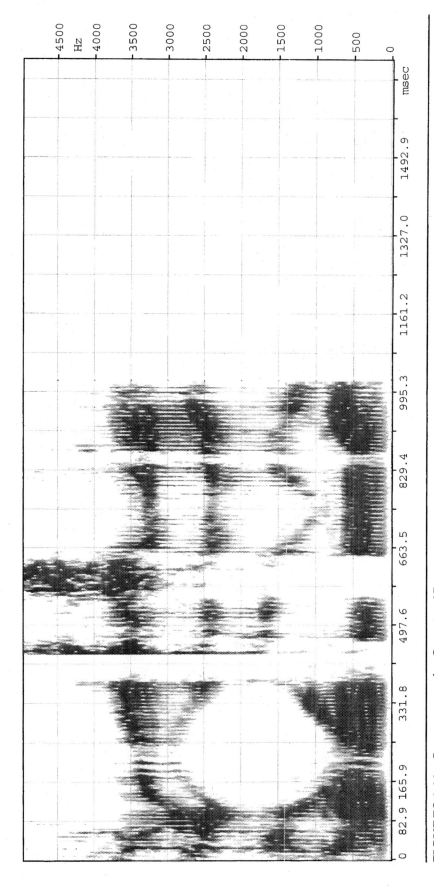

FIGURES 9-28 Spectrogram for Question 3B.

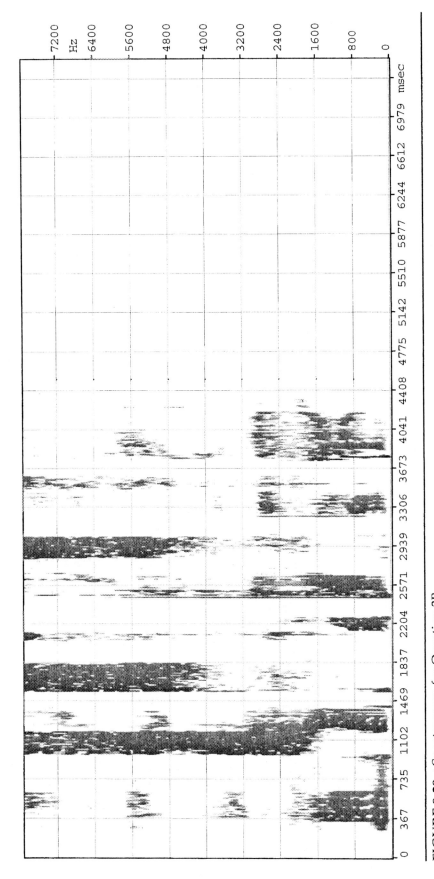

FIGURE 9-29 Spectrogram for Question 3B.

163

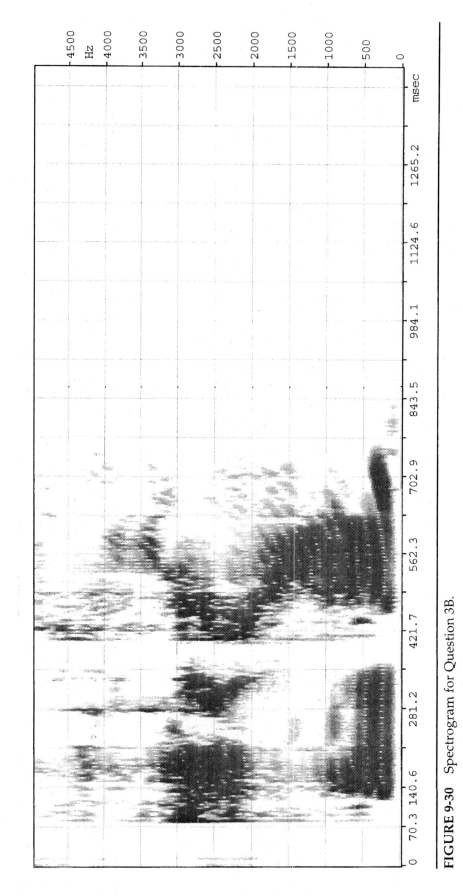

FIGURE 9-30 Spectrogram for Question 3B.

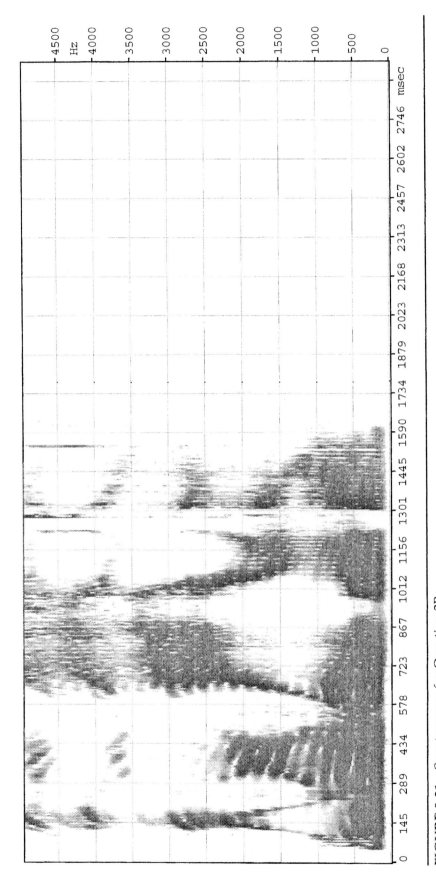

FIGURE 9-31   Spectrogram for Question 3B.

165

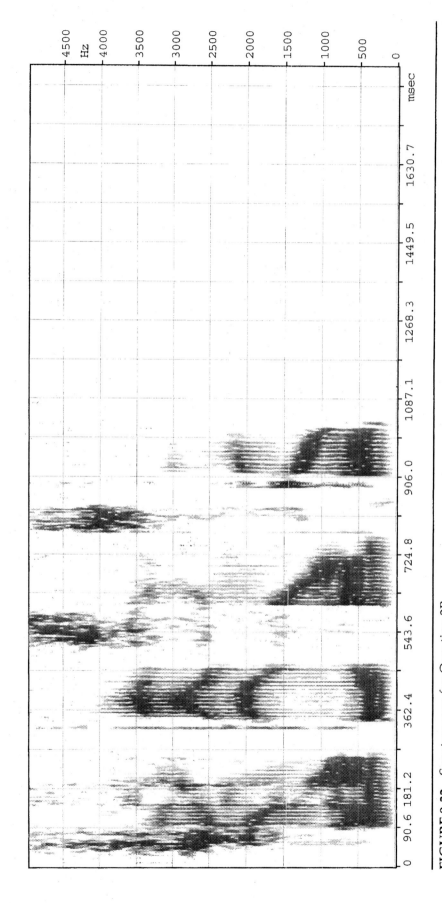

FIGURE 9-32 Spectrogram for Question 3B.

6. Which fricative has the lowest noise band frequency?

    a) [s]
    b) [v]
    c) [h]
    d) [θ]
    e) [ʒ]

7. Which fricative has the lowest noise band intensity?

    a) [s]
    b) [v]
    c) [h]
    d) [θ]
    e) [ʒ]

8. Formant frequencies are lowered when

    a) lip rounding occurs.
    b) air passes through the nasal cavity.
    c) the vocal cords are relaxed.
    d) b and c.
    e) a and b.

9. Voice onset time is shorter when

    a) a female speaks, in comparison to a male.
    b) a nasal is produced, in comparison to a liquid.
    c) [i] is produced, in comparison to [u].
    d) a voiced consonant is produced, in comparison to a voiceless one.
    e) none of the above.

10
Work and Energy

We began by discussing various properties of sinusoidal waves, namely wavelength, frequency, and propagation velocity, then extended these concepts to complex waves. This led to detailed treatment of speech production and speech recognition. Now we are going to start moving toward a detailed discussion of hearing. In order to understand the process of hearing, we must understand the wave property called amplitude. From the previous cursory treatment of wave energy (see second paragraph of Chapter 4, and Chapter 5, 5-A), you should realize that the energy carried by a wave is intimately tied to the amplitude of the wave. Since the energy of the wave is related to how loudly we hear a sound, amplitude is therefore related to loudness. We start our detailed discussion of wave energy by considering the concept of energy in physics.

10-A. Work and Energy

We begin by defining "work" as it is used in physics. Before providing the definition, however, you should be warned not to confuse the physics definition with the colloquial use of the word "work." The definition of "work" in physics is a precise statement about forces and distances.

Work (W) is done when a **force** (push or pull, denoted by F) causes an object to move through a **distance** (D). Numerically, the amount of work done by a force on an object is equal to the product of the force applied and the distance that the object **moved in the direction of the applied force**. Mathematically this can be expresses as follows:

$$W = F \times D$$

Examples of work, according to this definition, are

a) Pushing a car. As long as the car rolls along when you push it, you are doing work on the car. If you push a car and it does not move, you are doing no work on the car, regardless of your effort, because D is zero.

b) Lifting a box. You do work on the box when you lift it because you provide a force and move the box through a distance to a new height. There is a force—the exertion you use to overcome the weight of the box—and a distance equal to the height to which you lift the box.

c) A bulldozer pushing dirt. The bulldozer does work on the dirt, since it pushes the dirt through a certain distance.

Note that, according to our definition, you do no work if the object you push or pull does not move.

The amount of work that a force performs on an object also depends on how the force is applied. For example, the angle between the line along which the force is applied to an object and the direction of motion of the object is important in computing the net work done on the object by that force. To illustrate, suppose that you are coasting along on your bicycle while wearing a backpack. You are exerting a force vertically upward on the backpack to counteract its weight and keep it from falling. However, your motion is horizontal, so the distance the backpack moves is also horizontal. Because the force you are applying (directed upward) is perpendicular to the direction of motion (forward), by the physics definition of work, you do not do any work on the backpack.

● ANSWER THIS

In which of the following situations is work being done according to the physics definition of work?

a) A parachutist is in free fall after jumping out of an airplane. Does the gravitational force of Earth do work on the parachutist?

b) You lift a heavy box from the floor until your arms are extended and the box is above your head. Did you do work on the box?

c) You now hold the same heavy box over your head with your hands and walk horizontally for 10 meters. Did you do work on the box during your walk?

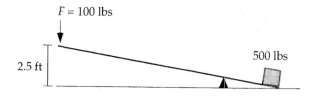

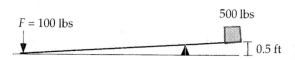

FIGURE 10-1 Using a lever to obtain mechanical advantage. The diagram shows how a 500-lb box can be lifted by a 100-lb force. Notice that the 100-lb force does work equal to $W = (100 \text{ lbs}) \times (2.5 \text{ ft}) = 250$ ft-lbs, and this work went into lifting the box 1/2 foot, since $(500 \text{ lbs}) \times (0.5 \text{ ft}) = 250$ ft-lbs.

The work done on an object also depends on whether a mechanical device is used to move it. For example, if you want to lift a 500-pound box, but you are capable of exerting only 100 pounds, you will not find it possible to lift the box directly. However, by using a lever (a lever works on the same principle as the seesaw) you can lift the weight, as shown in Figure 10-1. Devices like the lever, the pulley, the inclined plane, and the screw can be arranged to give you what is called "mechanical advantage"—that is, they can act like force magnifiers. As Figure 10-1 shows, the 100-pound force must act through a longer distance so that the work it does equals the work done to lift the 500-pound box.

Now we are ready for a definition of energy. **Energy** is the ability or capacity to perform work. It should be clear that there must be some relationship between work and energy. The work-energy theorem in physics relates work and energy, and we will discuss it later in this chapter. First it is useful to mention various forms of energy.

Kinetic energy is energy associated with motion. Two examples of bodies possessing kinetic energy are a thrown ball and a moving car. The formal mathematical definition of kinetic energy is

$$\text{kinetic energy} = (1/2) \times (\text{mass}) \times (\text{velocity})^2$$

where the mass and the velocity are those of the moving object. Note that since the kinetic energy depends on both the mass and the velocity, it is possible for a massive object moving at a small velocity to have the same kinetic energy as, or more kinetic energy than, a less-massive object moving at a high velocity.

Potential energy is energy that is stored and can be converted to kinetic energy, or to work, at some later time. Sometimes potential energy is associated with the position of an object. Some examples of potential energy follow.

a) An object suspended above the Earth on a rope (see Figure 10-2). An object that is at some height above the ground has potential energy relative to the ground that is given by the mathematical relationship

$$\text{potential energy} = (\text{weight}) \times (\text{height})$$

If the rope is cut, the object loses potential energy because it loses height as it drops. The **po-**

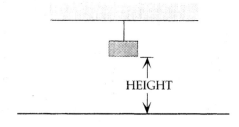

FIGURE 10-2 A box hanging at some height above the ground has potential energy, or energy of position. This potential energy is converted to kinetic energy if the string is cut. As the box loses height, thereby losing potential energy, it gains kinetic energy.

tential energy is converted to energy of motion, or kinetic energy, as the object falls. The factors in the potential energy equation are a force (the weight) and a distance (the height), which is the same as the factors in the definition of work. This is no coincidence, and we will see shortly how this type of energy is related to work.

Weight is related to **mass**. An object's mass measures the amount of material in the object and is the same wherever the object sits, whether on earth, on the moon, or in space where there is no gravity. Mass is a measure of the inertia in a body; the more massive an object is, the harder it is to accelerate, that is, to get it moving. That would be true anywhere in the universe; it is not dependent on gravity. Mass is measured in kilograms. An object's weight, on the other hand, depends on where it is in the universe. For example, if the object is on Earth, Earth's gravity pulls on it. A 1-kilogram object weighs about 2.2 pounds on Earth, but it would weigh less on the moon, where the gravitational pull on the object is weaker because the moon is less massive than Earth. In the metric system, we measure force (and weight) in units called newtons. Each kilogram of mass weighs about 10 newtons on earth.

b) A compressed spring with an object attached at the end (see Figure 10-3). A spring that is compressed or stretched a distance d from its relaxed (or equilibrium) length has a potential energy given by the mathematical expression

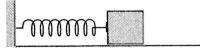

FIGURE 10-3   A stretched spring has potential energy. If the block is released with the spring stretched, the potential energy stored in the spring will be converted to kinetic energy of the block.

$$\text{potential energy} = (1/2) \times (k) \times (d)^2$$

where k is called the spring constant and is a number associated with the particular spring (stiff springs have large values of k, while loose or weak springs have small values of k). Suppose the spring shown in Figure 10-3 is stretched to the right so that d is large. If the object is released, the spring will give up its potential energy, and the object will pick up kinetic energy, that is, it will move to the left. (You might also think of an archer's bow as a spring that is stretched; the potential energy is transferred into the kinetic energy of the arrow.)

c) A dam holding back water. The water behind a dam can be allowed to fall over the dam, thereby converting potential energy into kinetic energy. The same mathematical expression given in example a) holds for the dam water, where the mass is the mass of the water that goes over the dam.

When viewed at a molecular level, the particles of an object will be observed to be in constant random motion. **Thermal energy** is the total of kinetic and potential energies involved with these random motions of the molecules. In a simple gas, the thermal energy

---

❀ ANSWER THIS

A diver comes off a diving board. What type of energy does she have at the highest point in her dive?

a) kinetic energy only

b) potential energy only, even if she is spinning at the top of her dive

c) potential energy only, but only if she is not spinning at the top of her dive

d) both kinetic and potential energy; it doesn't matter whether she is spinning at the top or not

e) none of the above

❀ ANSWER THIS

Which of the two objects in the following comparisons has more energy, and what type of energy is it?

a) a large truck parked on a level street, or a fluttering butterfly

b) a hot air balloon with three passengers on board descending at 5 feet per second, or a baseball thrown at 50 miles per hour

c) a 2-pound flower vase on top of a table, or a 50-pound box resting on the floor

is completely kinetic, and in this case, **temperature** is a measure of the average random kinetic energy of a molecule. An object with a higher temperature feels hotter. **Heat** is the thermal energy that is transferred from a hot object to a cold object because of their temperature differences. When two objects slide past each other with their surfaces touching, friction between the two surfaces will convert some of the kinetic energy of the objects into thermal energy (the frictional rubbing between the surfaces generates a heat flow, and the molecules of both objects end up with greater thermal energies and higher temperatures than prior to the rubbing).

10-B. Work-Energy Theorem

Work and energy are related by the **work-energy theorem,** which states that any change in the kinetic energy of a body is the result of having work done on it. This fundamental law establishes a formal relation between work and energy and enables us to define energy as the ability to do work. Of primary interest to us, however, is the **principle of conservation of energy**, which states that energy is neither created nor destroyed; it just passes from one form to another.

As an example of these concepts, let's consider a simple ideal mechanical system: a swinging pendulum. Figure 10-4 illustrates the position of a pendulum at various times. In a pendulum such as this, frictional losses would eventually turn all potential and kinetic energy into thermal energy; there is some friction at the pivot since the string rubs against the pivot as the pendulum swings, and the mass at the end of the string rubs constantly against air molecules since it is swinging in a "sea" of air. For the sake

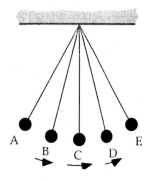

FIGURE 10-4   A simple pendulum. Notice the exchange between potential and kinetic energies as the pendulum swings.

of discussion, however, we will assume that there are no frictional losses (that is, that no kinetic or potential energy goes into other forms of energy, such as heat) so that the pendulum returns to the same height after every swing.

When at position A at the top of its swing, the pendulum's energy is all potential. As it moves down in its swing (from point A to point C), Earth pulls down on the mass and does work on it (in this case, positive work is done by Earth on the pendulum), thereby increasing its kinetic energy (according to the work-energy theorem). This increase in kinetic energy comes at the expense of potential energy. At the bottom of its swing at point C, all of the pendulum's energy is kinetic (we are assuming that height, which enters the equation for computing potential energy, is being measured from the bottom of the swing, so that potential energy is zero at the bottom of the swing). When the pendulum then swings up from C to E, the kinetic energy decreases while the potential energy increases. Because the pendulum's kinetic energy is changing (decreasing), according to the work-energy theorem, there must be some work being done on it; in this case, Earth does negative work on the pendulum, decreasing its kinetic energy. The decrease in kinetic energy is accompanied by an increase in potential energy, and at the top of its swing at point E, all of the pendulum's energy is again potential. Note a subtlety in this example: The string exerts a force on the pendulum, but it does no work according to the physics definition of the term. The force exerted by the string is always along its own length, toward the pivot point at the top. However, the pendulum never moves in that direction; the string always remains the same length. Only the gravitational force (neglecting friction) does work on the pendulum (both positive and negative work).

The ideal pendulum just described is called a **conservative system**, which means that the sum of potential and kinetic energies at any instant in time must be a constant value. That is, the sum of the kinetic and potential energies remains the same throughout the oscillations. The conservation of the sum of potential and kinetic energies for the pendulum is represented in graphical form in Figure 10-5. To get the sum of kinetic and potential energies at a given time, one adds the kinetic energy and potential energy at that time. The sum of kinetic energy and potential energy is always a constant value for all times, as shown by the long-dash horizontal line in Figure 10-5. Thus, even though the potential and the kinetic energies each vary as time passes, their sum remains constant.

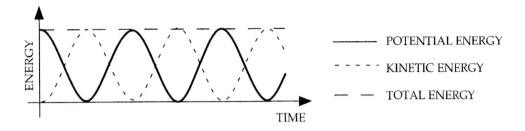

FIGURE 10-5 Potential energy (solid curve), kinetic energy (short-dash curve), and total energy (sum of the two, denoted by horizontal long-dash line) for a swinging pendulum. At time 0, the pendulum is released from rest at point A in Figure 10-4.

10-C. Wave Energy

Thus far, we have discussed different kinds of energies and the types of energies that a body can have. We have also discussed how the energy of one body can be transformed from one type into another, as in the pendulum example. Now we can begin to apply these concepts to waves.

Until now we have talked about a physical wave (e.g., a wave on a string or a sound wave) as a disturbance in a medium. The wave travels through the medium without causing any net transport of the material comprising the medium (there is no net movement of air volume as a sound wave propagates; the air molecules just oscillate back and forth). We have yet to discuss what physical property has been transmitted through the medium. When a wave is traveling through a medium, the **physical property that propagates through the medium is energy**. For waves on strings or sound waves, this propagation of energy must be in the form of either kinetic or potential energies (we are assuming an ideal world without friction by which thermal energy is generated). In most cases, the wave energy is a mixture of potential and kinetic energies all the time, although the nature of the mixture (the amount of kinetic and the amount of potential) varies with time.

A simplified model that displays how energy can travel through a medium and at the same time switch its form back and forth between kinetic and potential is a chain of masses connected to each other by "massless" springs. The top diagram in Figure 10-6 shows five masses connected by springs in their equilibrium positions. Starting in the diagram labeled A, a

longitudinal pulse is created by pulling the first mass toward the left and releasing it. The remaining diagrams depict the propagation of this hypothetical longitudinal pulse along the chain at various times. If we neglect friction, the total energy remains constant, although it is constantly changing form. For example, when mass 1 is moved to the left and released (as in diagram A), the energy is potential (stored in the springs connecting mass 1 to the wall and between masses 1 and 2). A little later, in diagram B, masses 1 and 2 are moving, and their interconnected springs are also stretched or compressed, so there is both kinetic and potential energies present. As time passes, subsequent diagrams (C–P) show how the pulse propagates toward the right. At any instant in time, the energy is distributed between kinetic (masses are moving) and potential (springs are stretched or compressed).

One way of telling what kind of energy is present in a wave at a particular instant in time is to consider whether parts of the medium are moving and whether parts of the medium are displaced from their usual or equilibrium positions. Recall that kinetic energy is energy of motion; thus, if the medium is moving, there must be some kinetic energy present in the wave. Also recall that potential energy is stored energy, so any portion of the medium that is displaced from its equilibrium position possesses potential energy.

As another example, let's consider the molecules of a traveling sound pulse in a solid (like a piece of metal) or a liquid (like water), as depicted in Figure 10-7.* Since some of the air molecules are displaced, some potential energy is present. Individual mole-

---

*The case of a sound pulse in a gas is not as simple as we discuss here. In a gas, the stored energy is not all potential, but rather due to increased random molecular motion in the regions of compression.

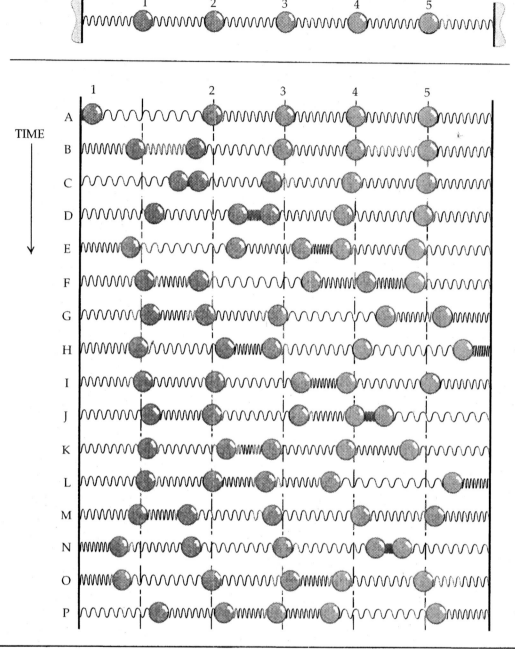

FIGURE 10-6 A hypothetical longitudinal pulse propagating down a chain of masses connected by springs. Note the interchange of potential and kinetic energies between springs and masses. From W. J. Leonard, R. J. Dufresne, W. J. Gerace, & J. P. Mestre, *Minds-On Physics: Complex Systems / Activities & Reader*, pp. R56–57. Copyright © 2001 by Kendall/Hunt Publishing Co., Dubuque, IA. Used with permission of Kendall/Hunt.

cules are moving within the medium so that there is kinetic energy present, just as in Figure 10-6. There is also a net velocity of the disturbance, say, to the right (although no permanent net transport of molecules from left to right takes place), so wave energy is transported from left to right. Further, there is thermal energy present because each molecule is undergoing random thermal motion, but again there is no net velocity in any given direction if we consider all molecules as a group. You can think of it as wave motion and thermal motion superimposed on each other.

As another example, consider a sinusoidal traveling sound wave produced by a loudspeaker that is creating periodic pulses, as shown in Figure 10-8. This

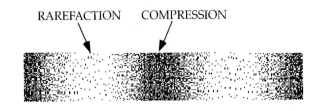

RAREFACTION   COMPRESSION

FIGURE 10-7 Model of the molecules in a traveling sound pulse in a solid or a liquid. Note regions of compression and rarefaction of molecules. The density variations are exaggerated for illustrative purposes.

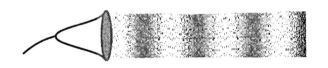

FIGURE 10-8 Model of a sinusoidal traveling sound wave generated by a loudspeaker. The dark regions correspond to compression of air molecules, while the light regions correspond to rarefaction of air molecules. The density variations are exaggerated for illustrative purposes.

situation is analogous to the individual pulse depicted in Figure 10-6, but now the loudspeaker is continuously generating a periodic wave (dark regions denote compressions; in between are rarefactions).

It should be evident that a traveling wave can be thought of as traveling energy. However, what about standing waves? Do they also consist of kinetic and potential energies? To answer this question, let's consider a string tied at both ends undergoing oscillations in its fundamental mode. This situation is shown in Figure 10-9 at four different instances in time.

The diagrams in Figure 10-9 suggest that a standing wave is also a combination of kinetic and potential energies. In picture A, the string has instantaneously come to a stop. Since there is no motion, there is no kinetic energy, but since the medium is displaced from its equilibrium position and the string is stretched (just as a spring is stretched), there is potential energy.** In picture B, all energy is kinetic since the string is certainly in full motion but the medium is not displaced, so there cannot be any potential energy. If we ignore friction, the total energy in the standing wave remains constant; that is, at any instant in time, the sum of the potential and kinetic energies is a constant value. In this sense, the standing wave example in Figure 10-9 is very similar to the pendulum in Figure 10-4.

10-D. Relation of Wave Energy to Wave Amplitude

To obtain a relationship between the amplitude of a wave and the energy of the wave, we will consider the oscillations of a block attached to the end of a spring, as shown in Figure 10-10. Let's assume that the spring is massless (that is, has very little mass in

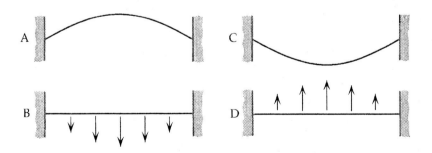

FIGURE 10-9 A string undergoing oscillations in its fundamental mode. In frames A and C, the string has come to rest momentarily and all of its energy is potential. In frames B and D, all of the string's energy is kinetic; in these two frames, parts of the string near the middle are moving faster than parts near the ends.

**The potential energy in this case is analogous to the energy stored in a stretched spring. Although there is also some gravitational potential energy in picture A since the string is higher than it would be in its equilibrium position, this is negligible in comparison to the stored energy from stretching.

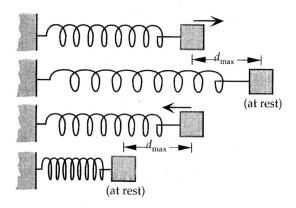

FIGURE 10-10 Oscillations of a block attached to a spring. Think of it as being on a slippery air table so that friction can be neglected. Note the exchange between potential and kinetic energies. In the first and third frames, all of the energy is kinetic, while in the second and fourth frames, all of the energy is stored as potential energy in the spring.

comparison to the block), and that the maximum distance that the spring stretches and compresses from equilibrium is d_{max}—in other words, the amplitude of the oscillations of the block on the spring is d_{max}. Further, we will assume that there is no friction, so that the block always oscillates in such a way that it reaches d_{max} on each oscillation.

This example is again analogous to the pendulum example in that the sum of potential and kinetic energies remains a constant value at all times during the oscillations. The energy does change form. When the block momentarily comes to rest at the instant that the spring is stretched or compressed a distance d_{max}, all energy is potential (kinetic energy is zero because the block is not moving) and is stored in the spring. When the block is moving at its maximum speed, all energy is kinetic because this occurs when the spring is in its equilibrium configuration (neither stretched not compressed). Since the total energy of the system does not change, we can compute this total energy at some convenient position, such as when the spring is maximally compressed and the block is momentarily at rest. At that instant, all energy is potential. The expression for this total energy is (see example b in Section 10-A)

$$\text{potential energy} = (1/2) \times k \times (d_{max})^2$$

Thus, we see that the total energy of this system goes as the square of the amplitude, d_{max}. The reason for this result is the elastic nature of the spring. When

you first try to compress or stretch the spring it is easy to do, but as you stretch it more you are pulling molecules in the metal farther apart, and the force necessary to accomplish this increases. Thus, the force needed to stretch (or compress) the spring is proportional to the displacement, $F = k \times d_{max}$, where k is still the spring constant. But the distance stretched is also d_{max}. Work is force times distance, and so that is proportional to $k \times d_{max} \times d_{max} = k\,(d_{max})^2$. (The factor $(1/2)$ is necessary in the potential energy formula because $k \times d_{max}$. is the maximum force that is applied; at the beginning only a weak force is necessary to stretch the spring, and it builds up to $k \times d_{max}$. The average force exerted is $(1/2)\,k \times d_{max}$.) We will find out later in this chapter that what we perceive as loudness is also related to the square of the amplitude.

10-E. Units of Energy

Before we can make quantitative statements about energy, we must agree on the units that we will use to measure it. Several different units are used to measure energy. In the English system, energy is measured in foot-pounds. As discussed in Section 10-B, energy and work are intimately related by the work-energy theorem; since work is defined as a force times a distance, it is easy to understand why these units apply—distance is measured in feet and force in pounds, so the product must have units of foot-pounds.

The system scientists prefer to use is the metric system. In this system, energy is measured in units called **joules** (named after James Prescott Joule, a famous physicist who showed that heat was another form of energy). One can easily convert foot-pounds to joules or vice versa by using the following conversion relationship: 1 foot-pound = 1.356 joules. One joule of energy is produced when one newton of force is exerted over one meter of distance. That is, a joule is also a newton-meter.

Let's make a few comparative statements about energy to get a feel for the units:

• One joule is the energy needed to lift a box weighing one pound a vertical distance of nine inches in Earth's gravitational field.

• A human weighing 165 pounds uses slightly over 220 joules to lift himself or herself one foot, and thus spends about 2200 joules climbing one flight of ten steps (assuming each step is about a foot).

• The energy released by a 100-watt lightbulb in 1 second is 100 joules. Hence, the work done by a person climbing a flight of steps is about the same as a 100-watt bulb burning for 20 seconds.

• One pound of coal, if completely burned, releases about 10 million joules.

• A small atomic bomb releases about 6 million million joules, which is equivalent to about 20,000 tons of TNT.

10-F. Relation of Energy to Power

Power is defined as the rate of doing work. The units of power, therefore, are energy per unit of time. In the metric system, power is measured in joules per second, or **watts** (one watt is one joule per second). A 100-watt lightbulb produces 100 joules of heat and light in 1 second; it produces 1000 joules in 10 seconds. A 50-watt lightbulb produces 50 joules in 1 second. However, if the 50-watt bulb is left on for 100 seconds, it will produce 5000 joules of energy, five times as much as the bigger bulb, simply because it was left on longer. The brightness of a standard incandescent bulb is dependent on the power of the bulb, the rate of energy production, not on the total energy produced. A 100-watt bulb is brighter than a 50-watt bulb. We will see that sound loudness also depends on power, not simply on total energy carried by the wave.

10-G. Relation of Power to Intensity

We have argued previously that the total energy of a sound wave remains constant, but that the spatial distribution of this energy can vary. For example, suppose we have a sound source generating sound waves in all directions. The wave fronts shown in Figure 10-11, which are drawn at distances d_1 and d_2 from the source, are spherical shells that contain the same total energy. However, since the wave front at distance d_1 is spread over a smaller spherical shell than the wavefront at d_2, the amplitude of the sound wave at position d_1 must be larger. In terms of hearing, this means that we would perceive the sound at distance d_1 as louder than the sound at d_2.

Thus, what we call the perceived loudness of a sound depends on the energy that reaches our ear per second, that is, the power of the sound source. Furthermore, as the diagram illustrates, the perceived loudness doesn't depend only on the power of the sound source because as we move farther from the source, the perceived loudness of the sound diminishes. Thus, perceived loudness depends on two factors: the power of the sound source and the surface

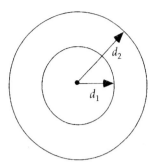

FIGURE 10-11 Depiction of two spherical wave fronts for a traveling sound wave. We would perceive the sound as louder at distance d_1 compared to d_2 since the total energy per second reaching our ears of the wave is spread over a smaller surface area at d_1 compared to d_2.

area over which this power is spread. What we perceive as loudness, therefore, is measured in terms of power per unit area.

The **intensity** of a sound is the power per unit area that reaches our ear, and it is intensity that we associate with loudness. In acoustics, intensity is measured in units of watts per square meter (W/m²). Following is a summary of the relationship between energy, power, and intensity.

• Energy is defined as the capacity to perform work. Its units are the same as the units for work, namely joules.

• Power is the rate at which work is done. It is measured in units of joules per second, which is called watts. Thus, power is energy per time.

• Intensity is what we perceive as loudness, and it is the power per unit area of a sound.

• Intensity is measured in units of watts per square meter, or equivalently, in joules per second per square meter.

Example: As an example, consider a standard incandescent lightbulb, call it A, that produces 1000 joules of energy in 20 s. This light is then concentrated by using a lens onto a spot that has an area of 0.0005 m². Another incandescent bulb, call it B, produces 100 W of energy in 2 s and this light is concentrated onto a spot of area 0.0002 m². Which spot appears brighter?

Solution: The brightness of the spot depends on the intensity. In the case of bulb A, the power is

1000 J/20 s = 50 W. The intensity is determined by dividing this by the area, or intensity of bulb A = $50W/0.0005m^2 = 100,000$ W/m². For bulb B the same calculation leads to an intensity of 100 $J/2s/0.0002$ m² = 250,000 W/m². Even though bulb B has produced less total energy, the spot produced by bulb B is brighter because that energy was concentrated in a shorter time and onto a smaller area.

Recall that the energy of a mass on a spring was proportional to the square of the amplitude; in the case of a wave, it is the energy per second per unit area that is proportional to the square of the amplitude. That is, the intensity of a wave, at some particular time and position, is proportional to the square of its amplitude: Intensity = (constant) × (amplitude)². The constant is a number that depends on the medium (on whether we are talking about waves on strings or in gases, as well as the type of string and the type of gas). To get a feeling for the meaning of this relationship for the energy carried by a wave, consider the following two cases: if you double the amplitude of a wave, you quadruple the wave's intensity; if you reduce the amplitude by a factor of three, then you reduce the wave's intensity by a factor of nine. Another way of expressing this formula is by writing:

$$I = I_0(A/A_0)^2$$

Where I is the wave's intensity when the amplitude is A, I_0 is the wave's intensity when the amplitude is A_0. Thus, if the amplitude of the standing wave on a string is increased from 2 inches to 6 inches, $A/A_0 = 3$ and $I = (3)^2 I_0 = 9I_0$. For sound waves, amplitudes measure pressure differences, so the intensity (or loudness) of a sound wave is proportional to the square of the pressure difference.

❂ ANSWER THIS

A musician playing a bass drum hits the drum softly, generating a pressure wave of amplitude A. A little later, the musician hits the drum very hard, generating a pressure wave having amplitude 2.5A. How much louder would the second sound be compared to the first?

10-H. Audible Levels of Intensity

The ear is a pressure-sensitive device. Our ears do not detect absolute pressure, but rather pressure fluctuations. We have seen how sound is really the propagation of pressure fluctuations. The ear is designed to nullify the effects of an overall change in pressure. The Eustachian tube, which connects the ear and the throat, balances pressure on both sides of the eardrum. Thus, only variations in external pressure cause the eardrum to vibrate. These vibrations are amplified and transmitted to the inner ear.

The flexible membrane called the eardrum does possess some physical limitations. If the intensity of a particular sound is too low, it will not be sufficient to move the eardrum (think of it as trying to get a bass drum to vibrate by hitting it with a very light feather). On the other hand, the eardrum has an elastic limit, and too intense a sound will cause it to vibrate with an amplitude large enough to rupture it (think of it as hitting a bass drum with a sledgehammer). Fortunately, intense sounds become painful to listen to before the eardrums reach this limit.

The range of intensities over which the ear is sensitive is extraordinarily large. The intensity of the faintest audible sound at 1000 Hz is

$$I_{min} = 0.000000000001 \text{ watts}/m^2$$

while the loudest tolerable sound is

$$I_{max} = 1 \text{ watts}/m^2.$$

Notice that the loudest sound we can tolerate still has a rather small intensity.

Given this large range of intensities over which our ears are sensitive, it is more convenient to express intensities in scientific notation, which involve powers of ten. Scientific notation is simply a convenient mathematical notation to express very small and very large numbers. This system of mathematical notation plays a major role in understanding and using the decibel scale of sound intensities, which we will study in the next chapter.

10-I. Scientific Notation (Powers of Ten)

As mentioned above, scientific notation is a convenient way to express numbers that take a lot of space to write down, such as 25,600,000,000,000, or 0.0000000985. Before we discuss how we would write these numbers, let's talk about powers of ten.

We can express any multiple of 10 as 10 raised to some power. For example, we can write

$$100 = 10^2.$$

The 2 in this equation is called an exponent, and the exponent simply tells you how many times you multiply the number by itself. In this case, the 2 means that you multiply 10 by itself, so another way to write the above equation is

$$100 = 10^2 = 10 \times 10.$$

You can read 10^2 as "ten squared" or as "ten to the second power." Other multiples of 10 expressed in scientific notation include

$$10 = 10^1 \text{ (ten to the first power)}$$
$$1000 = 10^3 = 10 \times 10 \times 10 \text{ (ten cubed, or ten to the third power)}$$
$$1000000 = 10^6 = 10 \times 10 \times 10 \times 10 \times 10 \times 10 \text{ (ten to the sixth power)}$$

Notice that the exponents are just the number of zeros when the number is written out longhand. So the number 10^{13} is equal to a 1 followed by 13 zeros.

Multiplying two multiples of 10 using scientific notation is simple. For example,

$$100 \times 100000 = 10000000 \text{ (longhand)}$$
$$10^2 \times 10^5 = 10^7 \text{ (in scientific notation)}$$

Notice that to multiply multiples of 10 using scientific notation, you add the exponents:

$$10^2 \times 10^5 = 10^{(2+5)} = 10^7$$

To divide multiples of 10 using scientific notation is also simple. For example,

$$1000000 / 100 = 10000 \text{ (longhand)}$$
$$10^6 / 10^2 = 10^4 \text{ (in scientific notation)}$$

To divide two numbers, subtract the denominator exponent from the numerator exponent:

$$10^6 / 10^2 = 10^{(6-2)} = 10^4$$

Since dividing two multiples of 10 in scientific notation involves subtracting their exponents, it is not unusual to end up with a negative exponent after a division. Let's now interpret the meaning of a negative exponent by looking at an example:

$$100 / 100000 = 1/1000 = 0.001 \text{ (longhand)}$$
$$10^2 / 10^5 = 10^{(2-5)} = 10^{-3} \text{ (in scientific notation)}$$

So we see that a negative exponent, say –3, means (one) divided by (ten raised to that exponent). Below are a few examples of tens with negative exponents and their decimal equivalents:

$$10^{-1} = 1/10^1 = 1/10 = 0.1$$
$$10^{-2} = 1/10^2 = 1/100 = 0.01$$
$$10^{-3} = 1/10^3 = 1/1000 = 0.001$$
$$10^{-20} = 1/10^{20} = 1/100000000000000000000$$
$$= 0.00000000000000000001$$

If you are given a decimal written in longhand, such as 0.00000001, and asked to write it in scientific notation, you should count the number of times that you need to shift the decimal point to the right until it is just after the digit 1, and that is the negative exponent needed:

$$0.\underset{\wedge\wedge\wedge\wedge\wedge\wedge\wedge\wedge}{0\,0\,0\,0\,0\,0\,0\,1} = 10^{-8} \} \text{ 8 shifts to the right, so the exponent is –8.}$$

You can also use this procedure for numbers greater than 1, only now count the number of times you need to shift the decimal point to the left until it is just to the right of the digit 1, and that is the exponent needed. For example,

$$1\,\underset{\wedge\wedge\wedge\wedge\wedge\wedge\wedge\wedge\wedge}{0\,0\,0\,0\,0\,0\,0\,0\,0}. = 10^9 \} \text{ 9 shifts to the left, so the exponent is 9.}$$

The final issue we will consider in this section is the meaning we should assign to ten to the zero power. We already know enough to deduce what the answer is. Let's consider the following division:

$$10000 / 10000 = 1 \text{ (longhand)}$$
$$10^4 / 10^4 = 10^{(4-4)} = 10^0 \text{ (in scientific notation)}$$

So you can see that ten to the zero power must be one.

10-J. Expressing Arbitrary Numbers in Scientific Notation

It is customary to write arbitrary numbers in scientific notation by starting with the first digit, followed by a decimal point, followed by however many digits follow the first digit, multiplied by the appropriate power of ten. This may sound confusing, but an example should illustrate the procedure:

$$543000 = 5.43 \times 100000 = 5.43 \times 10^5$$

Notice that we can use the same procedure used earlier. Count the number of places that you would need to shift the decimal point in order to move it to a position just to the right of the first digit, and this is the power of ten needed. Shifting the decimal point to the right results in a negative exponent, and shifting the decimal point to the left results in a positive exponent. Let's illustrate with some examples.

$$0.0000375 = 3.75 \times 10^{-5}$$
$$\text{^ ^ ^ ^ ^}$$

} five shifts to the right means an exponent of –5.

$$197. = 1.97 \times 10^2$$
$$\text{^ ^}$$

} two shifts to the left means an exponent of +2.

Don't simply memorize these rules blindly, because you are bound to mix them up. One sure way to check to see if the sign of the exponent is correct is to see whether you want the number multiplying the ten-raised-to-some-power to get bigger or smaller. For example, suppose you have the two cases,

$$6780000. = 6.78 \times 10^6$$

and

$$0.00000678 = 6.78 \times 10^{-6}$$

Notice that in the first case, you want to multiply 6.78 by a big number, namely 100,000, to get 6,780,000, so you would need a positive exponent to express large numbers like 100,000 in scientific notation. On the other hand, you need to multiply 6.78 by a small decimal, namely 0.000001, to get 0.00000678, and decimal numbers like 0.000001 require negative exponents when written in scientific notation.

10-K. Addition and Subtraction of Arbitrary Numbers in Scientific Notation

To add or subtract numbers expressed in scientific notation, you must make sure that the exponent of both numbers is the same before you add or subtract. For example, the following two numbers expressed in scientific notation can be subtracted immediately because they carry the same exponent:

$$\begin{array}{r} 6.56 \times 10^{12} \\ - 1.89 \times 10^{12} \\ \hline 4.67 \times 10^{12} \end{array}$$

However, these two numbers cannot be added or subtracted until you make both exponents the same:

$$\begin{array}{l} 2.03 \times 10^{-2} \\ + 1.80 \times 10^{-3} \end{array}$$ Change 1.8×10^{-3} to $(1.8 \times 10^{-1}) \times (10^1 \times 10^{-3}) = 0.18 \times 10^{-2}$.

Notice that all we did was multiply by 1 ($10^{-1} \times 10^1 = 1$) and regroup to change the power of 10 of the second number. Now both numbers have the same exponent, so you can add them:

$$\begin{array}{r} 2.03 \times 10^{-2} \\ + 0.18 \times 10^{-2} \\ \hline 2.21 \times 10^{-2}. \end{array}$$

By making the exponents the same, you guarantee that the appropriate digits are lined up in the proper columns with respect to the decimal point. In the example above, we didn't have to change the exponent of the second number; we could have left the second number alone, changed the exponent of the first number, and added the same two numbers as follows:

$$\begin{array}{r} 20.3 \times 10^{-3} \\ + 1.80 \times 10^{-3} \\ \hline 22.1 \times 10^{-3} = 2.21 \times 10^{-2} \end{array}$$

The same answer should result no matter which way you choose to do it.

10-L. Multiplication and Division of Arbitrary Numbers in Scientific Notation

To multiply two numbers expressed in scientific notation, multiply the "arbitrary-number" parts together and also multiply the "ten-raised-to-powers" parts together. You may need to re-express the answer in the appropriate scientific notation when you are done. Let's do two examples to see how this works.

$$(2.0 \times 10^3) \times (4.13 \times 10^{-2}) = (2 \times 4.13) \times 10^{(3-2)}$$
$$= 8.26 \times 10^1$$

$$(6.1 \times 10^{12}) \times (3.0 \times 10^2) = (6.1 \times 3) \times 10^{(12+2)}$$
$$= 18.3 \times 10^{14} = 1.83 \times 10^{15}$$

Use the same procedure for division.

$$(2 \times 10^6)/(4 \times 10^2) = (2/4) \times 10^{(6-2)}$$
$$= 0.5 \times 10^4 = 5.0 \times 10^3$$

$$(6.03 \times 10^{-4})/(3.0 \times 10^2)$$
$$= (6.03/3) \times 10^{(-4-2)}$$
$$= 2.01 \times 10^{-6}$$

Be particularly careful when you divide by a number that has a negative exponent; in this case subtracting a negative exponent means you add it.

$$(2.55 \times 10^7)/(5 \times 10^{-3}) = (2.55/5) \times 10^{(7-(-3))} =$$
$$0.51 \times 10^{10} = 5.1 \times 10^9.$$

Exercises

1. In which situation is work done on the object denoted in bold type below?

   I) A **book** falls a distance of 1 meter through the air.

   II) A child pulls a **toy truck** with a string and moves it 8 feet.

   III) A skater glides 50 feet across the ice while holding his **partner** over his head.

   a) I only   b) II only   c) III only

   d) I and II   e) II and III   f) I and III

   g) I, II, and III

2. Four people are moving a piano up a ramp (see Figure 10-12). One is pulling the piano with a rope, another is pushing it directly up the ramp, and the remaining two are pushing the piano sideways to make sure it does not stray from a straight path up the ramp. Which of the workers does work on the piano?

   a) all of them

   b) workers 1 and 3 only

   c) workers 2 and 4 only

   d) worker 3 only

   e) worker 1 only

   f) none of them

3. A book is dropped from a table onto the floor. Relative to the floor, what type of energy does the book have when it is halfway down?

   a) kinetic energy only

   b) potential energy only

   c) both kinetic and potential energy

   d) none of the above

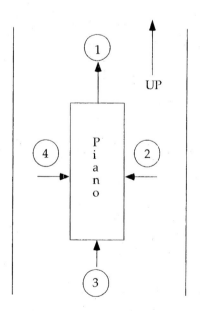

FIGURE 10-12 A piano is being moved up a ramp by four workers. Worker 1 pulls the piano with a rope; worker 3 pushes the piano; workers 2 and 4 push sideways to stabilize the piano. Assume that the piano moves along a straight line up the ramp.

4. A ball rolls down a ramp (see Figure 10-13). What type of energy does it have when it reaches the bottom of the ramp?

    a) kinetic energy only

    b) potential energy only

    c) both kinetic and potential energy

    d) none of the above

5. Figure 10-14 shows a standing wave in three positions of its cycle. Where in the cycle is the energy all kinetic energy?

6. How much work is done by a mother in carrying a 10-kg baby up a 6-meter-tall flight of stairs?

    a) 60 joules

    b) 600 joules

    c) cannot tell from information given

    d) none

7. Two standard incandescent lightbulbs are turned on for some period of time. Bulb A produces 100 joules of energy in 5 seconds. Bulb B produces 50 joules in 2 seconds. Which bulb is brighter?

    a) A

    b) B

    c) They are the same brightness.

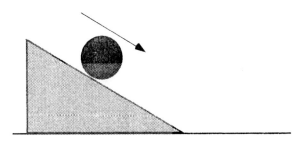

FIGURE 10-13   A ball rolling down a ramp.

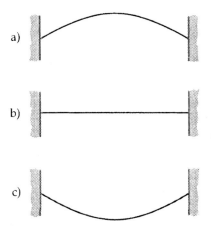

FIGURE 10-14   Choices for Question 5.

8. Bulb A from the previous question is concentrated to a spot of area 2 cm². Bulb B is concentrated to an area of 5 cm². Which spot is brighter?

a) A

b) B

c) Both are the same.

9. A sound wave has an intensity of 6 picowatts/cm². If its amplitude is tripled in size what is the resulting intensity? Note: One picowatt is 10^{-12} watts, and 10,000 cm² = 1 m².

a) 18 picowatts/cm²

b) 54 picowatts/ cm²

c) 108 picowatts/ cm²

d) none of the above

10. $10^2 \times 10^4 =$

a) 10^2

b) 10^6

c) 10^8

11. $36.7 \times 10^5 =$

a) 3.67×10^4

b) 3.67×10^5

c) 3.67×10^6

12. $0.283 \times 10^{-6} =$

a) 2.83×10^{-5}

b) 2.83×10^{-6}

c) 2.83×10^{-7}

13. $10^{-2}/10^{-6} =$

a) 10^4

b) 10^{-8}

c) 10^{-4}

d) 10^8

e) $10^{1/3}$

14. $7 \times 10^7 - 8 \times 10^6 =$

a) -1×10^1

b) -1×10^7

c) 6.2×10^7

d) 1×10^1

e) -1×10^{13}

15. $5 \times 10^{-3} + 0.3 \times 10^{-1} =$

a) 5.3×10^{-3}

b) 0.8×10^{-2}

c) 8.0×10^{-3}

d) 3.5×10^{-2}

11
Perception of Sound Intensity

We are now ready to discuss the scale used for measuring sound intensities. Intensities are measured in units of energy per time per area, and the favored set of units to use is watts per square meter (W/m^2). (Recall that the watt is a measure of power, which is energy per time.) It is customary to characterize any sound intensity by a ratio of that intensity to the intensity of the faintest audible sound at 1000 Hz. Thus we say that a particular sound has an intensity that is some multiple of the intensity of the faintest audible sound. To express this ratio as a convenient number, however, it is standard to consider the logarithm of the ratio rather than the ratio itself. Such a scale of intensity is known as the bel scale, where the usual unit of intensity is called the decibel. Learning to convert from watts per square meter to decibels requires us to review the use of logarithms and related mathematical topics.

A second main item covered in this chapter concerns the perception of loudness. Two sounds played at the same intensity but at different frequencies will not sound equally loud, because our hearing is more sensitive to certain frequencies than to others. For example, we will not hear a dog whistle at any intensity, because its frequency is completely beyond our range of hearing. Although loudness is a somewhat subjective experience, loudness levels can be quantified in terms of a unit called the phon. At any particular frequency, the phon scale can be related to the decibel scale.

11-A. The Bel Scale for Sound Intensities

As stated earlier the faintest audible sound at 1000 Hz, which we will denote as I_{min}, is

$I_{min} = $ (1 millionth) of (1 millionth) W/m^2

(W/m^2 means watts per square meter). In scientific notation, 1 millionth is 10^{-6}, so

$$I_{min} = 10^{-6} \times 10^{-6} \ W/m^2 = 10^{-12} \ W/m^2.$$

Also recall that the loudest tolerable sound intensity, I_{max}, is

$$I_{max} = 1 \ W/m^2.$$

When referring to sound intensities, rather than stating the absolute intensity level as a specific number of watts per square meter, it is customary to express intensities as a ratio. The ratio used is the intensity of the sound in question divided by the minimum audible intensity, I_{min}. For example, suppose we have a sound with intensity $I = 10^{-3} \ W/m^2$. The ratio that is customarily used to express this intensity level is

$$\frac{I}{I_{min}} = \frac{10^{-3} \ W/m^2}{10^{-12} \ W/m^2} = 10^{(-3-[-12])} = 10^9.$$

In the example, the sound is 10^9 times more intense than the minimum audible intensity.

The **bel scale** of measuring intensities makes use of the exponent of the 10 in the ratio of intensities, that is, the logarithm of the intensity ratio. In other words, a sound having absolute intensity of 10^{-3} W/m^2 has an intensity of 9 bels in the bel scale. As another example, let's find the intensity in bels of a sound having absolute intensity of $I = 10 \ W/m^2$:

$$\frac{I}{I_{min}} = \frac{10 \ W/m^2}{10^{-12} \ W/m^2} = 10^{(1-[-12])} = 10^{13}.$$

Since the exponent of 10 is 13, this sound has an intensity of 13 bels. Hence, the following equation defines the bel scale of sound intensities:

$$\frac{I}{I_{min}} = 10^{(\text{number of bels})}.$$

11-B. The Decibel Scale for Sound Intensities

Generally, the intensity of an arbitrary sound will not likely be expressible as a whole number of bels, but rather as a fractional number of bels. For example, a particular sound may have an intensity of 3.6 bels and another 8.5 bels. If we use the **decibel** scale (abbreviated as dB), we can avoid writing the decimal point that would be required to write intensities in bels. A decibel is one-tenth of a bel (the prefix, "deci," implies one-tenth of, just as "centi" implies one-hundredth of, as in centimeters). If one decibel is one-tenth of a bel, then there must be ten decibels in one bel. For example, an intensity level of 3.5 bels is 35 decibels, an intensity of 9.9 bels is 99 dB, and so on.

Table 11-1 gives a feel for the decibel scale by providing the intensity of various sounds in decibels.

TABLE 11-1 Comparison of Various Sounds in Decibels and in Watts per Meter Squared

Sound	Level in dB	Intensity (W/m²)
Hearing damage	140	10^{+2}
Large jet at takeoff	130	10
Threshold of pain	120	1
Chainsaw	110	10^{-1}
Lawnmower	100	10^{-2}
Noisy street	90	10^{-3}
Barking dog	80	10^{-4}
Conversation	60	10^{-6}
Home	50	10^{-7}
Quiet music	40	10^{-8}
Whisper	20	10^{-10}
Computer fan	10	10^{-11}
Threshold of hearing	0	10^{-12}

11-C. Fractional Powers of Ten

In Chapter 10, we considered integer powers of ten. To work with the decibel intensity scale, we will need to know how to deal with fractional, or decimal, powers of ten. In order to convert decibels to an absolute intensity measured in W/m², one must first convert decibels to bels, then figure out the value of ten raised to that many bels. For example, suppose that a sound has an intensity of 35 decibels, and you are asked to find the absolute intensity of this sound in W/m². The procedure to be followed is this:

a) Convert decibels to bels: 35 dB = 3.5 bels.
b) Use the definition of the bel scale to write:
$$\frac{I}{I_{min}} = 10^{3.5}.$$
c) Solve for the absolute intensity:
$$I = (I_{min}) \times 10^{3.5} = (10^{-12} \, W/m^2) \times 10^{3.5}$$
$$= 10^{-12+3.5} \, W/m^2 = 10^{-8.5} \, W/m^2.$$

As you can see, it is necessary to handle the fractional powers of ten here.

Although logarithms, as shown in the next section, are generally needed to deal with fractional powers of ten, we can use our knowledge of division and multiplication in scientific notation to deduce the meaning of decimal (or fractional) exponents. Consider what ten raised to the one-half power means (that is, 10 raised to the 0.5 power). Although the value of 10 raised to the 0.5 power may not be immediately obvious, we can see that if we multiply 10 raised to the 0.5 power by itself, we will get 10 because exponents add when multiplying. That is,

$$10^{0.5} \times 10^{0.5} = 10^{(0.5+0.5)} = 10^1 = 10.$$

Since $10^{0.5}$ multiplied by itself gives 10, then $10^{0.5}$ must be the square root of 10. That is,

$$10^{0.5} = \sqrt{10} = 3.16 \quad \text{(rounded off)}.$$

As another example, let's consider what would happen if we multiplied ten raised to the one-third power by itself three times:

$$10^{(1/3)} \times 10^{(1/3)} \times 10^{(1/3)} = 10^{(1/3+1/3+1/3)} = 10^1 = 10.$$

Ten raised to the one-third power is the cube root of 10:

$10^{(1/3)} = \sqrt[3]{10} = 2.15$ (rounded off).

One can deal with improper fractions, or decimals greater than 1, in the same fashion. For example,

$$10^{2.5} = 10^{(.5+2)} = 10^{.5} \times 10^2$$
$$= 3.16 \times 10^2 = 316 \quad \text{(rounded off)}.$$

and

$$10^{3.25} = 10^{(.25+3)} = 10^{.25} \times 10^3 = \sqrt[4]{10} \times 10^3$$
$$= 1.78 \times 10^3 = 1780 \quad \text{(rounded off)}.$$

11-D. Logarithms

We can now generalize from our discussion of fractional powers of ten to the concept of logarithm. The **logarithm** of some number, call it y, is the x in the equation, $10^x = y$ (x is the logarithm of y). Restated, the logarithm of y is the exponent, x, such that ten to the x power results in y. The logarithm of y, namely x, is written as follows:

$$x = \log(y).$$

Here is a useful alternative way of writing this equation:

$$10^x = 10^{\log(y)} = y.$$

A shorthand mnemonic is "the logarithm is the power of ten." As an example, we know from the previous section that 10 to the one-half power is approximately 3.16. Thus, according to the definition, the logarithm of 3.16 is 0.5 because 10 raised to the 0.5 power results in 3.16:

$$10^{0.5} = 3.16$$
$$\text{thus, } \log(3.16) = 0.5.$$

It is customary to abbreviate the word "logarithm" as "log." To find logs of arbitrary numbers, one can either consult a table of logarithms (Table 11-2) or use a scientific calculator. Looking up the logarithm of 8 in a mathematical table of logs or, equivalently, entering 8 in a scientific calculator and pressing the *log* button, results in 0.90309. Mathematically, this means that

$$10^{0.90309} = 8$$
$$\log(8) = 0.90309.$$

11-E. Logs of Products and Quotients

One of the major advantages of using logarithms is that all multiplication or division is performed by just adding or subtracting the logarithms. Suppose you want to multiply two numbers, A and B. In logarithm notation, this product can be written in the form:

$$A \times B = 10^{\log A} \times 10^{\log B} = 10^{(\log A + \log B)};$$

therefore,

$$\log(A \times B) = \log A + \log B.$$

The log of a product is the sum of the logs.

Similarly, to divide two numbers, A and B, you would get

$$\frac{A}{B} = \frac{10^{\log A}}{10^{\log B}} = 10^{(\log A - \log B)};$$

therefore,

$$\log\left(\frac{A}{B}\right) = \log A - \log B.$$

The log of a quotient is the difference of the logs.

Consider the logarithm of a number to a power, say,

$$\log(y^2) = \log(y \times y) = \log(y) + \log(y) = 2\log(y).$$

This result is general, that is, $\log(y^a) = a\log(y)$ for any power a. The logarithm of a power of a number is the power times the logarithm of the number.

11-F. Logs of Numbers Between 0 and 1, and Greater Than 10

Table 11-2 gives only the logarithms of numbers between 1.0 and 10.0. To find the log of a number greater than 10 without a calculator, first write the number in scientific notation, then take the log of the product, which you get by adding the logs.

TABLE 11-2   Logarithms of Numbers 1.0 to 10.0

N	Log N	N	Log N	N	Log N	N	Log N	N	Log N
1.0	0								
1.1	.0414	3.1	.4914	5.1	.7076	7.1	.8513	9.1	.9590
1.2	.0792	3.2	.5051	5.2	.7160	7.2	.8573	9.2	.9638
1.3	.1139	3.3	.5185	5.3	.7243	7.3	.8633	9.3	.9685
1.4	.1461	3.4	.5315	5.4	.7324	7.4	.8692	9.4	.9731
1.5	.1761	3.5	.5441	5.5	.7404	7.5	.8751	9.5	.9777
1.6	.2041	3.6	.5563	5.6	.7482	7.6	.8808	9.6	.9823
1.7	.2304	3.7	.5682	5.7	.7559	7.7	.8865	9.7	.9868
1.8	.2553	3.8	.5798	5.8	.7634	7.8	.8921	9.8	.9912
1.9	.2788	3.9	.5911	5.9	.7709	7.9	.8976	9.9	.9956
2.0	.3010	4.0	.6021	6.0	.7782	8.0	.9031	10.0	1.0
2.1	.3222	4.1	.6128	6.1	.7853	8.1	.9085		
2.2	.3424	4.2	.6232	6.2	.7924	8.2	.9138		
2.3	.3617	4.3	.6335	6.3	.7993	8.3	.9191		
2.4	.3802	4.4	.6435	6.4	.8062	8.4	.9243		
2.5	.3979	4.5	.6532	6.5	.8129	8.5	.9294		
2.6	.4150	4.6	.6628	6.6	.8195	8.6	.9345		
2.7	.4314	4.7	.6721	6.7	.8261	8.7	.9395		
2.8	.4472	4.8	.6812	6.8	.8325	8.8	.9445		
2.9	.4624	4.9	.6902	6.9	.8388	8.9	.9494		
3.0	.4771	5.0	.6990	7.0	.8451	9.0	.9542		

Example 1: Find log(730).

Solution: $\log(730) = \log(7.3 \times 10^2) = \log(7.3) + \log(10^2)$

From the table of logs, the log of 7.3 is 0.863. The log of 10^2 is just the exponent, 2. Therefore, the log of 730 is log (730) = 0.863 + 2 = 2.863 (which means that $10^{2.863} = 730$).

Example 2: Find log (0.0056).

Solution: $\log(0.0056) = \log(5.6 \times 10^{-3}) = \log(5.6) + \log(10^{-3})$

From the table of logs, the log of 5.6 is .748; the log of 10^{-3} is −3, so the answer is log(0.0056) = 0.748 − 3 = −2.252 (which means that $10^{-2.252}$ = 0.0056).

To find the log of a number between 0 and 1, first write the number in scientific notation, then take the log of the product.

The log of any of these numbers can also be obtained using a scientific calculator by entering the number and pressing the *log* button. In Example 2, entering 0.0056 and pressing the *log* button would result directly in –2.252.

11-G. *Logs and Negative Numbers*

Note two important properties of logarithms. First, logarithms are not defined for negative numbers. One cannot write log(–6), because there is no way to raise 10 to any power to get a negative number. (Don't confuse this with raising 10 to a negative power, which is a legal operation and will result in a number between 0 and 1, that is, a decimal fraction.) If you attempt to take the log of a negative number using a scientific calculator, the calculator's display window will notify you that an error has occurred.

Second, the logarithm itself can be a negative number. Numbers that lie between 0 and 1 always have negative logarithms. See Example 2.

❉ Answer This

Find the logarithms of the following numbers

a) 1,000   b) 8   c) 4.8   d) 3.5×10^{-2}
e) 2000   f) 500,000   g) $2.1 \times 10^{-2} \times 4.0 \times 10^{6}$
h) 0.00032   i) 438×10^{5} j) $5 \times 10^{-3} / 2 \times 10^{3}$

The following are logarithms (the power of ten representation) of some numbers. Find the numbers.

a) x   b) 2   c) 4.8   d) 0.5
e) –0.5   f) –16.5

11-H. *Some Examples Involving Decibels*

In this section we work out several examples involving the decibel scale. Instructions are given for working the problem either by longhand with the table of logs, or by using a scientific calculator.

Example 3: Convert the intensity, $I = 2 \times 10^{-6}$ W/m², to both bels and decibels.

Solution:

Using the table of logs

a) Apply the definition of the bel scale.

$$\frac{I}{I_{min}} = 10^{(\text{number of Bels})}.$$

b) Substitute the values for I and I_{min} in the equation above.

$$\frac{2 \times 10^{-6}\,W/m^2}{10^{-12}\,W/m^2} = 2 \times 10^{-6+12}$$
$$= 2 \times 10^{6} = 10^{(\text{number of bels})}.$$

c) Take the log of both sides, and use the rule for taking the logs of products.

$$\log(2 \times 10^{6}) = \text{number of bels}$$
$$[\log 2 + \log 10^{6}] = \text{number of bels}$$
$$0.301 + 6 = \text{number of bels}$$
$$6.301 = \text{number of bels}.$$

d) To convert bels to decibels, multiply the number of bels by ten.

$$\text{number of decibels} = 10 \times 6.301$$
$$= 63 \text{ (rounded off)}.$$

Thus, an intensity of 2×10^{-6} W/m² corresponds to an intensity of 6.3 bels or equivalently to an intensity of 63 decibels.

Using a scientific calculator

a) Apply the definition of the bel scale.

$$\frac{I}{I_{min}} = 10^{(\text{number of bels})}$$

b) Substitute the values for I and I_{min} in the equation above.

$$\frac{2 \times 10^{-6}\,W/m^2}{10^{-12}\,W/m^2} = 10^{(\text{number of bels})}.$$

c) Compute the quotient on the left-hand side in step b by hand or with your calculator.

$$\frac{2 \times 10^{-6}\,W/m^2}{10^{-12}\,W/m^2} = 2 \times 10^{6} = 10^{(\text{number of bels})}.$$

d) Use your calculator to take the log of 2×10^6, which is equal to the number of bels. (To take the log of 2×10^6 with your calculator, enter the number, 2×10^6, and press the *log* key.)

$$\log(2 \times 10^6) = \text{number of bels}$$

$$6.301 = \text{number of bels}.$$

Example 4: An acoustic architect is trying to measure the sound intensity of a particular sound in a large hall. The architect uses a microphone with surface area of 2×10^{-4} square meters, and the sound energy measured over a 4-second interval is 3×10^{-8} joules. Find the intensity of this sound in decibels.

Solution: a) First convert the data to an intensity measured in watts per square meters. To do this, recall that power is the rate of using energy. Since the microphone detected a certain amount of energy measured in joules over a certain period of time, we can find the number of watts as follows.

$$\text{power} = \text{energy/time} = (3 \times 10^{-8} \text{ joules})/ (4 \text{ seconds}) = 7.5 \times 10^{-9} \text{ W}.$$

The intensity is the power per unit area; thus we have

$$I = (7.5 \times 10^{-9} \text{ W})/(2 \times 10^{-4} \text{ m}^2)$$
$$= 3.75 \times 10^{-5} \text{ W/m}^2.$$

Proceed just as in Example 3 to find the number of decibels.

b) Apply the definition of the bel scale.

$$\frac{I}{I_{\min}} = 10^{(\text{number of bels})}.$$

c) Substitute the values for I and $I_{\min}$ in the equation above.

$$\frac{3.75 \times 10^{-5} \text{ W/m}^2}{10^{-12} \text{ W/m}^2} = 3.75 \times 10^7 = 10^{(\text{number of bels})}$$

d) Take the log of both sides (either with a calculator, or using the rule for taking logs of products).

$$\log(3.75 \times 10^7) = \text{number of bels}.$$

$$7.57 = \text{number of bels}.$$

e) To convert bels to decibels, multiply the number of bels by ten.

$$\text{number of decibels} = 10 \times 7.57 = 75.7 \text{ dB}.$$

Example 5: What is the intensity in W/m^2 of a 48-decibel sound?

Solution:

a) First convert 48 dB to 4.8 bels.

b) Then apply the definition of the bel scale.

$$\frac{I}{I_{\min}} = 10^{4.8}.$$

c) Solve for I.

$$I = I_{\min} \times 10^{4.8}$$
$$= (10^{-12} \text{ W/m}^2) \times (10^{4.8}).$$

With a calculator, you may now use the y^x key to find the value of $10^{4.8}$. To do so, enter 10, press the y^x key, then enter 4.8, press =, and the answer, 63095.73, should appear in the calculator's display screen. The answer is then

$$I = (10^{-12} \text{ W/m}^2) \times (10^{4.8})$$
$$= (10^{-12} \text{ W/m}^2) \times (63095.73)$$
$$= 6.31 \times 10^{-8}.$$

If you don't have a calculator, the longhand way to proceed is to express the product above as follows.

$$I = (10^{-12} \text{ W/m}^2 \times (10^{4.8}) = (10^{-12} \text{ W/m}^2) \times (10^4) \times (10^{0.8}).$$

If we know what 10 to the 0.8 power is, we can simply multiply the three numbers to obtain the answer. To determine the value of $10^{0.8}$ without a calculator, we use the table of logs in reverse. This is called taking an **antilog**. Look in the table under the log N entries and find the number closest to 0.8. The entry closest to 0.8 is 0.7993, which corresponds to 6.3. Hence, 6.3 must be 10 to the 0.8 power. Substituting and multiplying out we obtain the same answer as before:

$$I = (10^{-12} \text{ W/m}^2) \times 10^4 \times 6.3 = 6.3 \times 10^{-8} \text{ W/m}^2.$$

11-I. *Intensity Level versus Loudness Level*

The physical quantities inherent in a sound wave, such as frequency and intensity level, are properties of the wave itself and can be measured independent of any human. In contrast, the subjective properties of waves, such as pitch and loudness, are judgments made by an individual listener. This brings us to the distinction between intensity level and loudness level. Whereas intensity level is an objective physical property of a sound wave and can be measured by electronic instruments in W/m^2, bels, or decibels, loudness level is a subjective quality. Nevertheless, psychoacoustic experiments have allowed the development of a subjective scale for measuring loudness level. This scale uses units called **phons**. Just as decibels are the objective units used to measure intensity level, phons are the subjective units used to measure loudness level.

A typical experiment to determine loudness levels goes as follows. Earphones are placed on an individual, and two different pure tone frequencies are played on each ear. One ear receives a 1000 Hz note at various intensity levels. The other ear receives a different pure tone frequency, and the individual is asked to change the intensity level of this tone until it is at the same loudness as the 1000 Hz tone. When the data are analyzed, the results reveal that our judgment of loudness is not the same at all frequencies. For example, a 200 Hz tone at an intensity level of 40 dB is perceived as being at the same loudness as a 1000 Hz tone at 20 dB. Since both of these sounds are perceived at the same loudness, they both correspond to the same number of phons. The phon scale is related to the decibel scale by setting the number of phons equal to the number of decibels of an equally loud sound at 1000 Hz. On this scale, the 200 Hz tone with an intensity level of 40 dB has a loudness level of 20 phons, because the equally loud sound at 1000 Hz has an intensity of 20 dB.

The graph in Figure 11-1 shows the phon con-

tours as a function of frequency and is known as a **Fletcher-Munson diagram**. The contours show all sounds that are perceived to be at the same loudness level; thus all points, for example, on the 40 phon contour would sound equally loud, but their corresponding intensity levels, shown on the vertical scale at the left vary greatly as the frequency is changed. The loudness level of a tone at 1000 Hz is always equal to the intensity level of that tone measured in dB, in accord with definition of the phon scale.

A few examples will illustrate how the graph on page 192 is used:

Example 6: What is the intensity level of a pure tone played at 100 Hz that has a loudness level of 10 phons? (Another way to ask this same question is: What must be the intensity level of a 100 Hz pure tone in order for it to sound just as loud as a 1000 Hz tone played at 10 dB?)

Solution: To answer the question, look at the 10 phon contour and find where it meets the vertical line corresponding to 100 Hz; you now read the decibel reading off the left vertical axis to be about 45 dB.

Example 7: What is perceived as louder, a 100 Hz tone played at 60 dB or a 10,000 Hz tone played at 60 dB?

Solution: From the table, find the 60 dB intensity level on the leftmost vertical axis, and look horizontally across to where the 100 Hz vertical line crosses it. You can see that this point is midway between the 30 and 40 phon contours, so let's approximate the loudness level of this sound as 35 phons. Now find the 60 dB intensity level on the left and trace it across to where the 10,000 Hz vertical line crosses it. You can see that this point lies between 40 and 50 phons, but that it is much closer to the 50 phon contour. Approximate its loudness level as 48 phons. Therefore, because the loudness level (48 phons) of the 10,000 Hz tone at an intensity of 60 dB has a larger value than the loudness level (35 phons) of the 100 Hz tone played at same intensity level, the 10,000 Hz tone sounds louder.

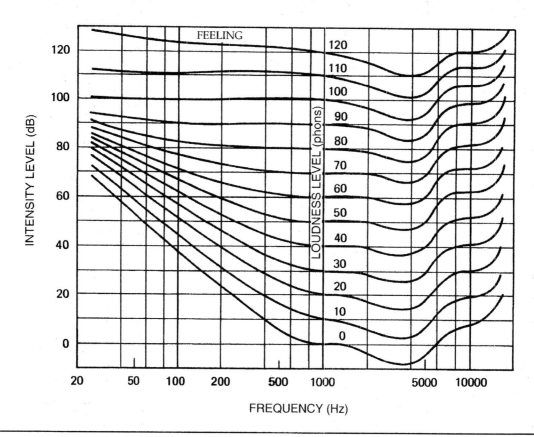

FIGURE 11-1 The Fletcher-Munson diagram showing loudness level contours in phons on an intensity versus frequencies plot. Sounds at all frequencies along any contour have the same loudness level. The corresponding intensity level is shown on the vertical scale. The phon level and the intensity level in dB are identical at 1000 Hz. From F. N. Martin and J. G. Clark, *Introduction to Audiology*, 7E © 2000, Reprinted by permission of Allyn & Bacon.

Example 8: What must be the intensity level of a 500 Hz tone in order for it to be perceived at the same loudness as a 10,000 Hz tone played at 90 dB?

Solution: Find the 90 dB intensity level on the left, and trace it across to where it intersects the 10,000 Hz vertical line. Notice that you are almost on top of the 80 phon contour. To have the same loudness, the 500 Hz tone must also have a loudness level of 80 phons. So follow the 80 phon contour to 500 Hz, and read across to find the intensity level of 80 dB.

Example 9: Assume that a 100 Hz tone and a 1000 Hz tone both are at an intensity level of 100 dB. Notice from the graph that, at this intensity, these two tones are both on the 100 phon contour, so they would sound equally loud. Now reduce the intensity levels of both tones by 50 dB. What is the difference in the loudness level of these two tones, measured in phons?

Solution: At the start, both tones are at 100 phons. When you reduce the intensity level by 50 dB, the 1000 Hz tone goes to 50 phons, while the 100 Hz tone goes to about 18 phons. Thus the 1000 Hz tone sounds about 32 phons louder than the 100 Hz tone when they are both at an intensity of 50 dB. (This means that when you reduce the volume on your stereo, the low-frequency tones are perceived to be considerably less loud than the high-frequency tones. To compensate for this, you would have to turn up the bass knob. Some sound systems will compensate for this if you just push a loudness button.)

✸ **ANSWER THIS**

What is the intensity level in dB of a 200 Hz tone with a loudness level of 50 phons?

What is perceived as louder, a 100 Hz tone played at 51 dB or a 10,000 Hz tone played at 30 dB?

11-J. *Negative Decibel Values*

The loudness graph also indicates that decibel values can be negative. For example, find the 0 phon contour at frequencies in the range 2000–4000 Hz. Notice that the contour dips below 0 dB. This means that, at these frequencies, a person with normal hearing can hear below the so-called threshold of audibility, I_{min}, which corresponds to 10^{-12} W/m², or equivalently, to 0 decibels. The next example shows you how negative decibel values come about.

Example 10: A 3000 Hz tone having intensity I = 3×10^{-13} W/m² is played. What is the intensity level of this tone in decibels?

Solution: First apply the definition of the bel scale by taking $\dfrac{I}{I_{min}}$, and setting it equal to $10^{(\text{number of bels})}$:

$$\frac{I}{I_{min}} = \frac{3 \times 10^{-13} \text{ W/m}^2}{10^{-12} \text{ W/m}^2} = 10^{(\text{number of bels})}.$$

Now take the log of both sides to get:

$$\log (3 \times 10^{-1}) = \text{number of bels}$$
$$0.477 - 1 = \text{number of bels}$$
$$- 0.523 = \text{number of bels}.$$

The number of decibels is 10 times this, or –5.23 decibels.

A negative decibel value simply means that the intensity of the sound is below the minimum intensity, 10^{-12} W/m². In a range of frequencies between 1200 Hz and 6000 Hz, someone with normal hearing (typically a young person) can detect sounds below the so-called threshold of audibility, I_{min}. As we will find in the next chapter, this extra sensitivity arises from a resonance and amplification of sounds in the ear canal.

11-K. *The Addition of Intensity and Loudness*

Suppose that two pure tones are played together, one having frequency 1000 Hz and the other having frequency 100 Hz. Further, suppose that both tones individually have an intensity of 20 dB. What would be the intensity of the combined tone? *Warning:* What might seem like the obvious answer, namely 40 dB, which is obtained by simply adding the two intensity levels, would be wrong. It is not correct to find the total intensity of two or more pure tones sounded together by simply adding up the individual decibel levels of all the tones, because adding decibels means that you are adding the exponents of the intensity, not the intensity themselves. What must be added are the intensities in Watts per square meter.

The following steps need to be followed to find the total decibel level of a combination of pure tones, each played at specific intensities.

a) Begin by changing the decibel level to bels.

b) Express the intensity in terms of I_{min} times 10 to the appropriate power (that is, 10 raised to the number of bels) by application of the definition of the bel scale.

c) Add the intensities, since they are expressed in watts per square meter, and write your answer in terms of I_{min} times the appropriate number expressed in scientific notation.

d) Finally, convert the result back to decibels.

Examples show how this procedure works.

Example 11: We return to the problem posed at the beginning of this section. What is the total decibel level of a 100 Hz tone and a 1000 Hz tone, each having an intensity level of 20 dB, if they are played together?

Solution:

a) First change the 20 decibels of either tone to 2 bels.

b) Next, express this intensity in terms of I_{min} times 10 to the 2 bel power by applying the definition of the bel scale.

$$\frac{I}{I_{min}} = 10^{(\text{number of bels})} = 10^2.$$

Solve for I:

$$I = 10^2 \times I_{min}.$$

c) Since both tones have the same intensity level, the total intensity level is obtained by adding two of these intensities.

$$I_{combined} = (10^2 \times I_{min}) + (10^2 \times I_{min})$$
$$= 2 \times 10^2 \times I_{min}$$

d) Convert this to bels and then to decibels.

$$\frac{I_{combined}}{I_{min}} = 2 \times 10^2 = 10^{(number\ of\ bels)}.$$

Take the log of both sides to get the number of bels.

$$\log (2 \times 10^2) = number\ of\ bels$$

$$0.301 + 2 = 2.301 = number\ of\ bels.$$

Thus, the combined tone has an intensity of 2.3 bels, or 23 decibels.

Adding two tones, each having an intensity of 20 decibels, results in an increase of only 3 decibels over the intensity of one of the single tones. This increase of 3 decibels when doubling an intensity is general for any initial intensity, not just for the 20 dB level. It arises from the fact that $\log(2)$ is very close to 0.3.

Example 12: Find the total intensity in decibels when you play the following three tones together: 300 Hz at 30 dB, 1000 Hz at 50 dB, and 3000 Hz at 40 dB.

Solution:

a) The intensities in bels of these three tones are 3, 5, and 4 bels, respectively.

b) You can write the three intensities as I_{min} times 10 to the appropriate power by applying the definition of the bel scale.

$$\frac{I_{300}}{I_{min}} = 10^{(number\ of\ bels)} = 10^3 \text{ or } I_{300} = 10^3 \times I_{min},$$

$$\frac{I_{1000}}{I_{min}} = 10^{(number\ of\ bels)} = 10^5 \text{ or } I_{1000} = 10^5 \times I_{min}$$

$$\frac{I_{3000}}{I_{min}} = 10^{(number\ of\ bels)} = 10^4 \text{ or } I_{3000} = 10^4 \times I_{min}.$$

c) Add up the three intensities.

$$I_{tot} = I_{300} + I_{1000} + I_{3000} = (10^3 + 10^5 + 10^4) \times I_{min}$$
$$= (1.11 \times 10^5) \times I_{min}.$$

d) Convert back to decibels.

$$\frac{I_{tot}}{I_{min}} = 1.11 \times 10^5 = 10^{(number\ of\ bels)}.$$

e) Finally, take the log of both sides to get the number of bels:

$$\log (1.11 \times 10^5) = number\ of\ bels$$

$$0.041 + 5 = 5.041 = number\ of\ bels.$$

The combined tone, therefore, has an intensity of 50.4 decibels. Note that the intensity of the combined sound is totally dominated by the tone having the largest intensity.

This same procedure can be used to add intensities when they are given as loudness levels. However, phons must be converted to decibels before the intensities can be added. Example 13 illustrates this point.

Example 13: What is the total intensity level (in dB) of a 100 Hz tone and a 1000 Hz tone, each having a loudness level of 70 phons, if they are played together?

Solution: Before we can apply the first step, we need to convert the phon levels to decibels. A 1000 Hz tone at a loudness level of 70 phons has an intensity level of 70 dB by definition. The 100 Hz tone at 70 phons has an intensity level of about 78 dB. Now we are ready to add these two intensities.

a) The intensity in bels of these two tones is 7 and 7.8.

b) Write the intensities in terms of I_{min}.

$$\frac{I_{1000}}{I_{min}} = 10^{(number\ of\ bels)} = 10^7 \text{ or } I_{1000} = 10^7 \times I_{min},$$

$$\frac{I_{100}}{I_{min}} = 10^{(number\ of\ bels)} = 10^{7.8} \text{ or } I_{100} = 10^{7.8} \times I_{min}.$$

c) Add the two intensities.

$I_{tot} = (10^7 + 10^{7.8}) \times I_{min} = (10^7 + [10^{(.8 + 7)}]) \times I_{min}$

$\qquad = (10^7 + [10^{.8} \times 10^7]) \times I_{min}.$

(Use a calculator, or the log table to obtain $10^{.8} = 6.3$.)

$\qquad = ([1 \times 10^7] + [6.3 \times 10^7]) \times I_{min}.$

$\qquad = 7.3 \times 10^7 \times I_{min}.$

d) Convert back to decibels.

$$\frac{I_{tot}}{I_{min}} = 7.3 \times 10^7 = 10^{(\text{number of bels})}.$$

Take the log of both sides to get the number of bels.

$$\log (7.3 \times 10^7) = \text{number of bels}$$

$$0.86 + 7 = 7.86 = \text{number of bels}.$$

The combined tone has an intensity of 78.6 decibels, which is pretty near the intensity of the 100 Hz tone. Again, notice the domination of the tone having the larger intensity.

❖ ANSWER THIS

Five sound sources, each at an intensity of 10^{-2} W/m², are combined. What is the dB level of the combined sounds?

11-L. *Notes on Reference Levels*

The decibel was defined in terms of the ratio of the sound intensity I to $I_{min} = 10^{-12}$ W/m², the approximate least audible sound intensity, by the formula

$$\text{sound level (dB)} = 10 \log\left(\frac{I}{I_{min}}\right).$$

The reference level chosen is convenient and commonly used, but it is not the only one possible. The decibel level quoted for a sound is often followed by a set of letters that tell the reader precisely what reference level has been used for the particular intensity quoted. Thus, for example, a sound having intensity 10^{-11} W/m² would be found from the formula to have a level of $10 \log(10^{-11}/10^{-12}) = 10$ dB IL. The "IL" (standing for intensity level) tells the reader explic-

itly that the reference level used was $I_{min} = 10^{-12}$ W/m².

Another equivalent, but much more common notation, is often used. Recall from Chapter 10 that intensity is related to amplitude, which for a sound wave is the maximum pressure change in the wave, which we will call P. But intensity is proportional, not just directly to P, but to P^2. (See Section 10-G.) That is, $I = C P^2$ where C is a constant not depending on the amplitude. From this result we could write our formula as

$$\text{sound level (dB)} = 10 \log\left(\frac{CP^2}{CP_R^2}\right) = 10 \log\left(\frac{P^2}{P_R^2}\right)$$

where C has canceled out and P_R is reference value for the pressure. The reference level used in most sound-level meters is $P_R = 20 \times 10^{-6}$ Pascals (Pa), which is more often written as 20 μPa (μPa means microPascal, or 10^{-6} Pa). Atmospheric pressure is about 10^5 Pa, so sounds correspond to very small pressure differences. This standard is very close to the pressure amplitude in a sound wave having an intensity of 10^{-12} W/m². However, to make absolutely clear that the pressure P_R is the reference level rather than I_{min}, sound levels using this scale are denoted as "dB SPL," where "SPL" stands for sound pressure level.

Because of the relation $\log (y^a) = a \log(y)$ (see Section 11-E), we can write

$$\text{sound level (dB SPL)} = 10 \log\left(\frac{P^2}{P_R^2}\right) = 20 \log\left(\frac{P}{P_R}\right).$$

Example 14: A sound of intensity 10^{-10} W/m² is found to have a pressure amplitude of 200 μPa. Compute the sound level in dB IL and dB SPL.

Solution: The sound level in dB IL is

$$10 \log\left(\frac{10^{-10}}{10^{-12}}\right) = 10 \log\left(10^2\right) = 20 \text{ dB IL}.$$

The sound level in dB SPL is

$$20 \log\left(\frac{200}{20}\right) = 20 \log\left(10^1\right) = 20 \text{ dB SPL}.$$

Note that the resulting decibel level is exactly the same, although in principle there could be very small differences.

Exercises

1. Find the logarithm of 2,100,000.

   a) 5.3222
   b) 6.3222
   c) 2.1×10^6
   d) 6.0
   e) none of these

2. Log x = 1.6021. What is x?

   a) 5.1
   b) 40.0
   c) 2.1×10^6
   d) 6.0
   e) none of the above

3. Find the logarithms of the following numbers.

   a) 6
   b) 4.5
   c) 2.1×10^2
   d) 5,100,000
   e) 265
   f) 162×10^{12}
   g) 21×10^{-6}
   h) 2000
   i) .00064

4. Below are the logarithms of some numbers. Find the value of the numbers.

   a) log y = 2.4
   b) log x = 0.8
   c) log z = 9.3
   d) log r = –0.32
   e) log w = –11.82

5. Convert the following intensities to decibels.

   a) $I = 3.7 \times 10^{-6}$ W/m^2
   b) $I = 2.1 \times 10^{-10}$ W/m^2
   c) $I = 10^{-17}$ W/m^2

6. Several measurements are taken in a concert hall with electronic equipment. The data recorded by five different meters are shown below. Which meter recorded the greatest intensity level?

   a) Meter 1: Area = 1 cm^2, 2×10^{-8} joules measured in 1 second
   b) Meter 2: Area = 1 cm^2, 3×10^{-8} joules measured in 2 seconds
   c) Meter 3: Area = 2 cm^2, 4×10^{-8} joules measured in 2 seconds
   d) Meter 4: Area = 3 cm^2, 3×10^{-8} joules measured in 2 seconds
   e) Meter 5: Area = 4 cm^2, 6×10^{-8} joules measured in 1 second

7. Add the following pairs of intensities to find the approximate total dB level. All sounds are made by a 1000 Hz tone. The set of choices apply to all three problems. Can you find the answers without doing any math?

A. 30 dB added to 30 dB   B. 50 dB added to 10 dB   C. 70 dB added to 65 dB

a) 71 dB

b) 33 dB

c) 60 dB

d) 40 dB

e) 50 dB

8. Which sound is louder, 100 Hz tone at 70 dB or 10,000 Hz tone at 55 dB?

9. What must the intensity level of a 100 Hz tone be so that it sounds as loud as a 1000 Hz tone at 65 dB?

10. A 100 Hz tone at 40 phons is played simultaneously with a 1000 Hz tone at 60 phons. What is the total intensity of the combined sound?

a) 40 dB

b) 60 dB

c) 64 dB

d) 100 dB

e) 120 dB

11. A 100 Hz tone at loudness 40 phons is played simultaneously with a 1000 Hz tone at intensity 40 dB. What is the intensity in W/m^2 of the combined sound?

12. Suppose the reference level for the decibel scale were set at $10^{-14} W/m^2$ (instead of the usual $10^{-12} W/m^2$). What would the decibel level for a sound having intensity of $10^{-11} W/m^2$ be?

a) −3 dB

b) −30 dB

c) 3 dB

d) 30 dB

e) 140 dB

12

The Ear and the Hearing Mechanism

In this final chapter, we discuss some aspects of the hearing mechanism, by which sound waves (pressure fluctuations) are received, amplified, mechanically transformed, and converted into electrical signals that proceed up the auditory nerve from the ear to the brain. We concentrate our attention on the mechanical part of conversion and do not discuss in any detail how the electrical signals are transmitted to or processed by the brain. The subject of this chapter is still being researched, and many properties of the hearing mechanism are not yet completely understood. Moreover, some of the processes apparently used by the ear involve physical effects whose discussion is beyond the level of this book, since it uses advanced mechanics, electrical network theory, or biology. Nevertheless, the elementary analysis given here should enable some basic insights into the nature of this amazing sensory organ.

The mechanical conversion of sound energy involves multiple steps wherein the energy is transferred through the three regions of the ear: the outer ear, the middle ear, and the inner ear. Figure 12-1 shows a diagram of the whole ear. We discuss each of the regions in turn. In our analysis of the inner ear, we will discover the existence of a wave unlike any discussed previously, the traveling wave on the basilar membrane.

12-A. The Outer Ear

The outer ear consists of the **pinna,** or **auricle,** which is the part that you can actually see, and the **ear canal,** or **external auditory meatus,** which terminates at the **eardrum,** or **tympanic membrane.** The pinna of the outer ear serves two functions. It captures and channels sound signals to the ear canal, and it helps us distinguish sounds originating directly in front of us from sounds originating behind us.

The meatus or ear canal is an air-filled passage about 28 mm long (a bit more than an inch) terminating at the eardrum. The ear canal serves as an acoustic resonator that can actually magnify pressure differences corresponding to its resonant frequencies. To illustrate how this happens, consider, as a model of the ear canal, an air tube open at one end and closed at the other. From our previous study of this type of air tube, we know that only certain wavelengths and frequencies are resonated in such an air column. The allowed frequencies (i.e., normal modes) are (see Section 3-D)

$$F_n = \frac{nv}{4L}$$

where v is the velocity of sound in air; $n = 1, 3, 5, \ldots$; and L is the length of the tube. Thus, the first resonant frequency for this model of the outer ear can be obtained by substituting $L = 28$ mm $= 0.028$ m, $n = 1$, and $v = 1100$ ft/s $= 335$ m/s:

$$F_1 = \frac{335 \text{ m/s}}{4 \times 0.028 \text{ m}} = \frac{335 \text{ m/s}}{0.11 \text{ m}} = 3045 \text{ Hz.}$$

Note that this first resonant frequency of the ear canal corresponds well to the range of frequencies where the ear is maximally sensitive, as shown in the Fletcher-Munson diagram in Figure 11-1—that is, where the 0 phon contour dips below 0 decibels.

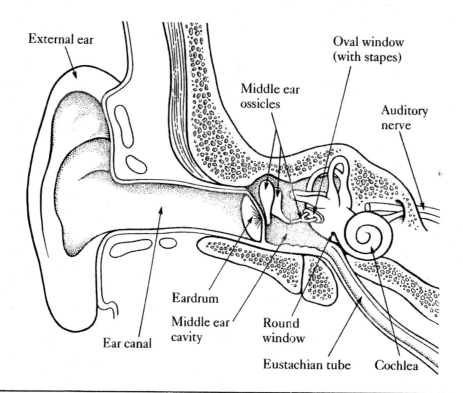

FIGURE 12-1   View of the ear, consisting of the three parts, outer or external ear, middle ear, and inner ear or cochlea. From: *The Speech Chain* by Peter B. Denes and Elliot N. Pinson © by W. H. Freeman and Company. Used with permission of Worth Publishers.

This model of the outer ear is somewhat crude because the ear canal is not a uniform tube; the canal is slightly tapered, with the wider end toward the outside. Also, the eardrum is a flexible membrane, not a rigid wall. Nevertheless, this model predicts the frequency range where the ear will be maximally sensitive. The function that the ear canal plays as a resonator makes it possible for us to detect sounds that would be imperceptible were the eardrum located at the surface of the head. Fortunately, the ear is not so efficient a resonator that it prevents other frequencies besides precisely the resonant one from penetrating to the ear drum. The ear canal also protects the eardrum from physical damage.

12-B. *The Middle Ear*

The middle ear cavity contains three small bones called the **ossicles** (Figure 12-2). The three ossicles consist of the **hammer** or **malleus**, which is attached on one side to the eardrum and on the other side to the second bone, called the **anvil** or **incus**. This in turn is attached to the third bone, called the **stirrup** or

stapes, whose other side covers the **oval window**, which is the entrance to the inner ear. The part of the stapes that covers the oval window is called the **footplate** of the stapes. The function of these bones is to transmit the vibrations of the eardrum to the fluid of the cochlea in the inner ear.

The ossicles function as an impedance matching device, a term explained below. To appreciate fully the ingeniousness of this mechanism, it is important to understand the reflection of waves at the boundary between two differing media. Recall (see Section 1-J) that when a traveling wave pulse on a string encounters a boundary, part or all of it is reflected. The pulse is reflected both when the medium becomes less dense after the boundary, and when it becomes more dense after the boundary. The reflection is complete only when the density after the boundary is either infinite (as for a string tied to a wall), or zero (as for a string whose end is free to move). In most instances, there is partial reflection and partial transmission of a wave when it encounters a different medium, as illustrated in Figure 1-18. Although we developed these ideas for waves on a string, they hold for sound waves in air and other media as well.

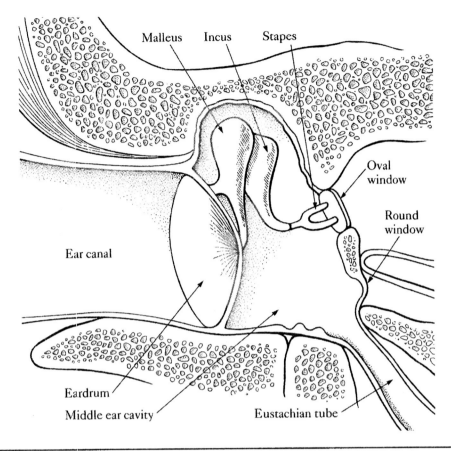

Malleus   Incus   Stapes

Oval window

Round window

Ear canal

Eardrum

Middle ear cavity

Eustachian tube

FIGURE 12-2   The middle ear. The ossicles, consisting of malleus, incus, and stapes, transmit sound from the ear drum to the inner ear. From: *The Speech Chain* by Peter B. Denes and Elliot N. Pinson © by W. H. Freeman and Company. Used with permission of Worth Publishers.

The term **impedance** is, in the case of waves, a measure of the resistance to the flow of wave energy. The impedance of a medium depends on three parameters: the elasticity (springiness), density (inertia), and friction of the medium. The density of a gas is its mass per unit volume; the density of a string is its mass per unit length. Elasticity measures how stiff an elastic medium is; for example, a big car spring is very stiff and hard to compress or stretch, while a small screen-door spring is less so. Differences in friction in a material can be seen in comparing a super-ball with a ball of putty. The superball loses very little energy in a bounce because it has so little internal friction, while a ball of putty hardly bounces at all because friction absorbs all the kinetic energy during a collision with the floor. Suppose a person uses his hand to get a wave started on each of two differing very long strings. If the mass density of one is larger, it is harder to get the wave started because of the greater inertia. If one string is more elastic than the other (harder to stretch), starting the wave will again be more difficult. Finally, if one string is immersed in water rather than in air, friction is higher, and it again becomes more difficult to get a wave started than when the string is in air. What actually governs how much wave energy is reflected and how much is transmitted at a boundary between two media is the **impedance mismatch** across the boundary. The ratio of the impedances of the two media is a measure of the impedance mismatch and therefore a measure of how well energy is transmitted. If this ratio is close to 1, the two media are well matched, and little reflection of the wave occurs (most of the wave is transmitted).

Impedance is a complicated mathematical combination of all three of these items, but in the simplest case, where friction is not a factor, the impedance, Z, is given by

$$Z = \rho c$$

where ρ is the density and c is the velocity of sound in the medium. Since c depends on both elasticity and density, it turns out that

$$Z = \sqrt{\text{density} \times \text{elasticity}}.$$

If the impedance of the material in which the wave is initially traveling is Z_1 and the impedance in which it travels when it crosses the boundary is Z_2, then the intensity in material 2, I_2, is given in terms of that in material 1, I_1, by

$$I_2 = I_1 \frac{4R}{(1+R)^2}$$

where $R = Z_2/Z_1$ is the ratio of the two impedances. While we have not derived this formula, we can see whether it makes sense. If the two impedances are the same, the ratio $R = 1$, and we see that

$$I_2 = I_1 \frac{4}{(2)^2} = I_1$$

so there is no reflection. On the other hand, if material 2 is absent altogether so that material 1 has a loose end, then $R = 0$, and we see that $I_2 = 0$, so that all the energy is reflected, as we expect. Finally, if material 2 is a wall, its impedance is infinite and so is R. For very large R, the denominator in the I_2 equation gets bigger faster than the numerator since it is squared, and we get I_2 approximately equal to $I_1 (4/R) \rightarrow 0$. Again, all the energy is reflected, as we expect.

Example: The impedance of air is 4.15×10^2 kg s/m^2 and that of water is 1.44×10^6 kg s/m^2. What is the percentage of intensity that enters the water when a sound wave in air meets the air-water boundary?

Solution: The ratio of impedances is

$R = \dfrac{4.15 \times 10^2}{1.44 \times 10^6} = 2.9 \times 10^{-4}$. Thus the ratio of intensities is

$\dfrac{I_2}{I_1} = \dfrac{4 \times 2.9 \times 10^{-4}}{\left(1 + 2.9 \times 10^{-4}\right)^2} = 1.1 \times 10^{-3} = 0.1\%$. Only one one-thousandth of the sound-wave energy enters the water.

If we want to transmit a wave across a boundary between two media with little reflection, we need to match the impedances of the two parts as nearly as possible. If the two parts were made of identical materials, then $R = 1$, but that would be equivalent to no boundary at all, and, of course, there would be no reflection. However, there are ways to match impedances when the two media are very different. Suppose the part on the right (material 2) has higher density than the left part (material 1); the impedance might be matched by increasing the elasticity of the lighter left part, so that the product of density and elasticity is the same on both sides of the boundary. The two strings would then have equivalent impedances, even though they are made of very different materials, and again no reflection would take place.

There is an even trickier way of matching impedances. Suppose we insert an intermediate material between media 1 and 2, one that gradually changes from the first kind to the second kind. If two strings have the same elasticity but very different densities, one might interpose a string whose density changes slowly from the low value on the left to the high value on the right. As the wave progresses over this intermediate string, it never sees a sudden change, so that very little reflection takes place. A megaphone is an example of this method of gradual change. The sound emanating from the mouth is coming from an enclosed tube to the open air, and reflection certainly takes place at the lips. The situation is similar to a nearly loose end of a string, as we noted in Chapter 3. (The reflection at the lips allows standing waves in the vocal tract to form that are the formants of the spoken sounds.) But that reflection makes it more difficult to get the sound out to an audience, and the vocal system has to work hard. With a megaphone, the opening at the lips is gradually increased in size until it is quite wide at the end of the megaphone, making a better match with the open air. The megaphone changes the effective nature of the vocal tract, and the sounds coming out of the megaphone are a bit distorted.

The ossicles play a crucial role in matching the impedance between the air in the outer ear and the fluid in the inner ear. To see how important this role is, consider as a model a situation in which the middle ear does not exist. Such conditions can actually occur, of course, when a person is born without ossicles or has them removed, or if they are not working properly due, say, to a middle ear infection. Figure 12-3 illustrates the situation, in which a pressure wave in air strikes the oval window of the inner ear. Behind the oval window is the cochlea, which is filled

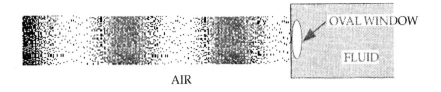

AIR

FIGURE 12-3   A schematic model of the ear without eardrum or middle ear. The sound wave, represented by the compressions traveling from the left, hits the oval window and must move the fluid inside the inner ear to produce a sensation of sound. A high percentage of the intensity would be reflected.

with a fluid having approximately the properties of seawater. Since the pressure wave encounters a different medium across the boundary (air on one side, fluid on the other), some of the wave energy will be reflected, and only a portion of it will be transmitted to the fluid in the inner ear. We see from the example above that only about 0.1 percent of the energy would be transmitted to the inner ear if a sound wave hit the oval window directly. The rest, or 99.9 percent, would be reflected. Thus, the ratio of the intensity transmitted to the intensity reflected is 0.1 to 99.9, or approximately .001= 10^{-3}. This means that if our ears were missing their middle sections, our hearing ability would diminish by 30 decibels (the exponent –3 of 10^{-3} represents 3 bels or 30 dB, and the minus sign means there is a decrease in sound intensity getting into the inner ear).

The fraction of the energy transmitted across the boundary can be increased by inserting an intermediate device to match the impedances across the two media. The impedance of a medium is also a measure of how much pressure must be applied to get the medium moving at a given velocity. The greater the impedance, the greater the pressure needed. Thus,

to avoid a large impedance mismatch, the pressure would have to be increased in the middle ear side of the oval window. This is precisely what the ossicles do.

This function of the middle ear of amplifying the pressure is performed by a combination of two physical principles: **lever action** and **area reduction**. The **lever** is a device, often just a steel rod or a stick, that enables one to enhance an applied force. The lever must be pivoted about a fulcrum, as shown in Figure 12-4. The figure shows how a 3 newton (N) weight can be lifted with a 1 N force, as long as the distance from the **fulcrum** (the pivot point) to the 1 N force is (at least) three times the distance from the fulcrum to the 3 N weight.

Note that you are not getting something for nothing since the work you put in is the work you get out. (See Section 10-A.) Recall that work is defined as the product of force times distance. If you push with a 1 N force and move the lever down a total distance of, say, 1.5 m, you have done 1.5 joules (J) of work on the 1 N weight. This means that the 3 N weight goes up only a distance of 0.5 m, since 3 N times 0.5 m is 1.5 J, which is exactly the amount of work you put in. In

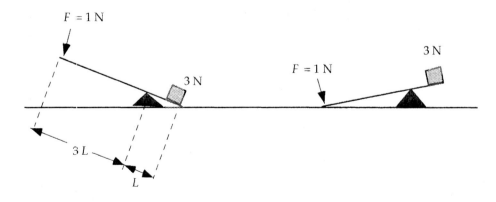

FIGURE 12-4   Lever action. A lever is a length of rigid material, such as a steel bar, that pivots about a fulcrum and allows a force on one end to result in a larger force on the other. In the case shown, a 3 N weight can be lifted by a 1 N force if the long lever arm is three times longer than the short arm.

short, a smaller force is applied (1 N), but it had to be applied over a larger distance (1.5 m) in order to get a larger force (the 3 N weight) to move over a smaller distance (0.5 m). Thus, the **amplification factor** of the lever shown below is 3 because the force applied, 1 N, is magnified threefold, allowing you to lift 3 N. Note that the amplification factor is also the ratio of the distances from the fulcrum to where the forces are applied.

⊛ **ANSWER THIS**

Explain how a simple bottle opener, such as the one on a Swiss army knife, acts as a lever. Where is the fulcrum in this case?

The ossicles of the middle ear act as a lever by which the force on the ear drum is amplified when applied to the oval window. There are ligaments at the front and back sides of the malleus and the incus that act as a fulcrum for rotation of the ossicles. The amplification factor of the middle ear due to lever action is not large—about 1.3. Recall that pressure is force per unit area, so that if the force is increased on a fixed area, the pressure is amplified as well.

The second form of pressure amplification by the middle ear is accomplished by area reduction. Since pressure is force per unit area, another way to amplify the pressure is to reduce the area over which the force acts. For example, suppose a cone-shaped object has 100 square centimeters (cm²) of surface area on one side and 10 cm² of surface area on the other (see Figure 12-5). If one applies a 200 N force at the left, the same force will be transmitted unchanged to whatever object stands to the right of the cone. However, the pressures on the right and left are very different. The pressure at the left is

$$P_{left} = (200 \text{ N})/(100 \text{ cm}^2) = 2 \text{ N/cm}^2.$$

The pressure at the right is

$$P_{right} = (200 \text{ N})/(10 \text{ cm}^2) = 20 \text{ N/cm}^2.$$

This situation illustrates how, for a given force, the pressure can be increased by applying the force over a smaller area. The effective area of the eardrum is about 19 times greater than the area of the stapes footplate; thus, the magnification that results from area reduction is about 19.

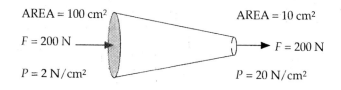

FIGURE 12-5　Pressure amplification. The force on the left is concentrated on the right on a smaller area, resulting in an increase in pressure on the right. Since the area is 10 times smaller on the right, the pressure is 10 times larger.

Thus, the force at the eardrum gets amplified by about a factor of 1.3 by lever action, and the area over which this force acts gets reduced by a factor of 19, resulting in an overall pressure amplification of about 25 (1.3 × 19). Finally, the intensity is proportional to the square of the pressure (as we saw in Chapter 10), so the ratio of the intensity of the inner ear to the intensity of the outer ear is 25^2 or about $625 = 10^{2.8}$. That is, the middle ear enables us to hear sounds whose intensities are about 625 times weaker than we could hear without it. This factor (an amplification of 28 dB) is almost what is needed to compensate for the transmission loss (30 dB) that would occur because of an impedance mismatch between the outer and inner ears. This means that a large fraction of the wave energy striking the eardrum is transmitted to the inner ear, available to be processed further.

An additional important point about impedance of the inner ear is that it changes with frequency. It is very large at low frequencies and is smallest at frequencies above 1500 Hz. At 100 Hz the ear transmits only about one-tenth of the energy transmitted at 1000 Hz. The result is that our hearing is less sensitive at low frequencies, as we saw in the diagram of Figure 11-1.

If the middle ear is not working properly, say, because an inflammation (otitis media) has caused fluid to fill the middle ear region or has blocked the Eustachian tube so it is unable to equalize pressure, sound will not be conducted well, and much of it will be reflected at the tympanic membrane. This factor is the basis of the operation of a device for detecting problems with the middle ear. This device, called an impedance audiometer, sends sound waves down the ear canal and detects how much is reflected. It does this as a function of external average air pressure in the canal; from the shape of the curve of impedance versus pressure, the operator can make a diagnosis.

Besides amplifying and transmitting sound signals, the middle ear also protects the inner ear from extremely loud sounds. This is accomplished by muscles attached to the eardrum and to the stapes. In response to loud sounds, the muscle attached to the eardrum pulls it in so it vibrates with less amplitude; at the same time, the muscle attached to the stapes pulls the stapes outward at the oval window. Both of these muscle actions reduce the middle ear's efficiency to transmit sounds. Yet another protective mechanism changes the axis of rotation of the stapes in a way that reduces the efficiency of transmitting forces.

> ❋ ANSWER THIS
>
> Explain how the bell on the end of a trumpet, trombone, or other brass instrument acts as an impedance matching device?

12-C. The Inner Ear

Our discussion has so far taken us two-thirds of the way through the ear. Sound waves in air travel down the ear canal and vibrate the eardrum. These vibrations are transmitted by the ossicles to the cochlea in the inner ear, which we next examine. Inside the cochlea, these mechanical vibrations are transformed into electrical impulses, which are sent to the brain.

Figures 12-1, 12-6, and 12-7 show the anatomy of the cochlea. It is a fluid-filled cavity shaped somewhat like a snail's shell, as seen in Figure 12-1. If we "unroll" it, as shown in Figure 12-6, it stretches about 35 mm from stapes to the apex. It is divided along its length by the cochlear partition, through which passes the **cochlear duct**. This latter is made up of several parts and can be seen in cross-section in Figure 12-7. The lower level of the partition is called the **basilar membrane**. On this rides the **Organ of Corti**, and attached to that is the **tectorial membrane**. The top partition is called **Reissner's membrane**. The end of the cochlea closest to the middle ear is called the basal end; the oval window, which is a membrane, is at the basal end, and the stapes rests on this window on the middle ear side. The oval window connects to the fluid in the **scala vestibuli**. The far end of the cochlea is called the **apex** or **apical end**. On the other side of the cochlear partition is the **scala tympani**. At the basal end of this chamber is the **round window**, which bulges out into the middle ear cavity when the oval window is pushed in, since the fluid in the cochlea is nearly incompressible. At the apex end of the cochlear partition is the **helicotrema**, an opening in the partition that allows fluid to pass from the scala vestibuli to the scali tympani.

Movement of the stapes transmits vibrations to the cochlear fluid, which in turn causes motions of the basilar membrane. The Organ of Corti resting on the basilar membrane contains **hair cells** that are connected to the tectorial membrane. There are about 16,000 hair cells throughout the cochlea. When the basilar membrane moves, these hair cells are bent, which causes them to generate electrical signals that are transmitted to the auditory nerve and sent as neural pulse patterns to the brain. The bending arises

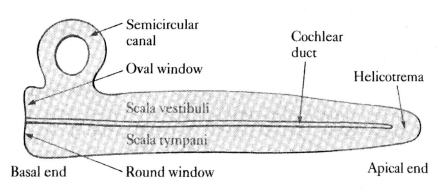

FIGURE 12-6 The cochlea unrolled to show the various segments in longitudinal section. From: *The Speech Chain* by Peter B. Denes and Elliot N. Pinson © by W. H. Freeman and Company. Used with permission of Worth Publishers.

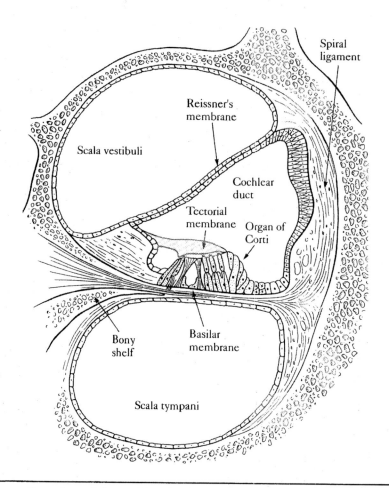

FIGURE 12-7   A cross section view of the cochlea. From: *The Speech Chain* by Peter B. Denes and Elliot N. Pinson © by W. H. Freeman and Company. Used with permission of Worth Publishers.

because the two membranes are pivoted on different axes so that a shearing force is placed on the hair cells when they move up or down, as illustrated in Figure 12-8.

In order for the brain to decipher speech and other sounds, it is necessary for it to disentangle the various frequency components and somehow make the equivalent of a spectrogram. Indeed, if loudness level is kept constant, the ear can distinguish about 1400 different frequencies. Near 1000 Hz, the ear can detect a change of about 3 Hz, a remarkable sensitivity to changes in frequency.

Understanding how the brain detects different frequencies has been the goal of hearing researchers for almost 150 years. The first real theory of hearing was suggested by Hermann von Helmholtz in a book in 1862. Helmholtz suggested that the cochlea contained the equivalent of a series of resonators, each of which was activated by an individual frequency component. A mechanical model of a device that acts somewhat like this is shown in Figure 12-9; a series of pendulums of differing length are hung from a rod. When the rod is oscillated at the natural frequency of one of these pendulums, that one will vibrate with the largest amplitude. The other pendulums will be out of resonance and will react with smaller amplitudes. Of course, one part of the basilar membrane is connected to the other and not made up of individual oscillators, but one could consider a more sophisticated model in which our pendulums are connected together loosely by small springs, and the results would not be changed much. While the Helmholtz theory is not quite right, it has considerable truth to it as we will see. An explanation like that of Helmholtz is called a **place theory** because frequency discrimination is associated with a particular place (the position of the resonator) in the cochlea. Such an idea has the advantage of allowing a complex wave

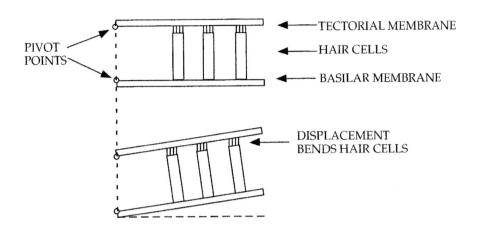

FIGURE 12-8   The hair cells are bent when the basilar and tectorial membranes are displaced because they are pivoted on different points. This bending converts mechanical energy into electrical energy that proceeds up the auditory nerve to the brain.

to be sorted out according to frequency along the cochlea.

An alternative model of the ear is a **volley** or **temporal theory**. One might conceive of the basilar membrane simply moving up and down with the frequency of an incoming sinusoidal wave and sending an electrical signal having the same number of pulses per second to the brain. It is a bit more difficult to model how such a system would decipher a complex wave into frequency components.

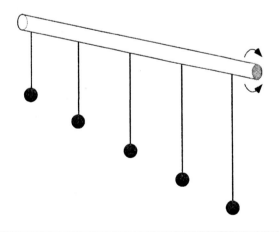

FIGURE 12-9   A series of pendulums all attached by strings to a rod that can make them swing when it is rotated. If the rod is rotated at the frequency of one of the pendulums, that one will have the maximum amplitude; the others, being out of resonance, will have smaller amplitudes.

The experimental research of Georg von Békésy starting in the 1920s was central to much of our understanding of the hearing mechanism. He showed that the basilar membrane varies in width and thickness along the cochlear partition. It is narrowest at the basal end, being only about 0.04 millimeters wide at that point. At the apical end, the membrane widens to about 0.5 millimeters. The membrane is thin and stiff (high elasticity) at the basal end and becomes thick and lax (low elasticity) at the apical end. What Békésy found, from working on cadavers and dead animals, was that a pure tone sent a **traveling wave** down the basilar membrane. The amplitude of this wave was not constant, but increased until it reached a maximum at a location that depended on the frequency. Beyond that point, the amplitude of the wave rapidly dropped to zero. The basic idea is that the place of maximum stimulation of the membrane and the hair cells near there correspond to the pitch we detect. For his work Békésy, won the Nobel Prize in 1961. Let's now look more closely at what is known about this process. The traveling waves set up have a behavior unlike any waves we have encountered previously.

Figure 12-10 shows a traveling wave set up on the basilar membrane. When the stapes pushes on the oval window, it is pushing on the fluid in the scala vestibuli, which is very hard to compress. This fluid pushes down on the basilar membrane. The basilar membrane, in turn, displaces the fluid in the scala tympani, which ultimately pushes out the round window. Just how and where the basilar membrane reacts maximally depends on the frequency of stimulation. At the basal end, the membrane is stiff and hard to

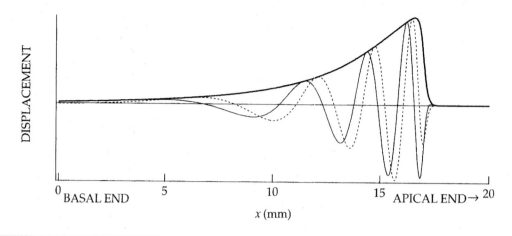

FIGURE 12-10   Displacement of the basilar membrane by a traveling wave set up when the stapes vibrates sinusoidally. The distance from the basal end is denoted as *x*, measured in millimeters. The entire basilar membrane is about 35 mm long. The light solid line is a snapshot of a wave. The dotted line is the same wave at a slightly later time, so that it is displaced to the right. The propagation velocity and wavelength decrease as the wave moves to the right onto less stiff parts of the basilar membrane. The main peak occurs at the region of the membrane that is in resonance at the frequency of the impressed wave. The amplitude diminishes rapidly to the right of that point. The heavy solid line is the envelope of the wave—that is, it traces out the positions that the maxima of the traveling wave sweep out. The figure is only qualitatively accurate. See the Web site for an animated version. ⊛

bend. The waves here will have high propagation velocity and long wavelength. As the traveling wave proceeds, it meets material of less stiffness, and the propagation velocity decreases. Note that in Figure 12-10, the peaks of waves at two differing times are closer together farther down the membrane, representing a smaller wavelength resulting from the smaller wave velocity. Furthermore, the membrane is less stiff here, so that a given pressure difference across the membrane from one scala to the other can produce a larger amplitude. This growth in amplitude and decrease in wave velocity continue until the point where the natural frequency of the oscillations of the basilar membrane match the frequency of the impressed sinusoidal wave. Here, as in all resonance phenomena, the amplitude is largest. Correspondingly, the wave velocity at this point has reached a small value, and the wave soon ceases to propagate. Any energy of the wave is absorbed in the friction of the fluid and membrane motion.

The point of resonance and maximum wave amplitude on the membrane depends on frequency. An easy way to illustrate this is to picture the envelope of the wave; this is the curve connecting all the points covered by the maxima of the wave as it travels from the basal end toward the apex. In Figure 12-10 the envelope is the dark solid line. Figure 12-11 plots the

envelope curves for various frequencies. It is apparent that the higher the frequency, the closer to the basal end the resonance occurs. Low frequencies have their maximum amplitude of traveling wave at the apical end. These results are expected because we know that the basilar membrane is stiffer at the basal end, so that its natural frequency there would be higher.

For most frequencies, the operation accords with a place theory of hearing. A complex wave will be separated into its components with high frequencies activating the basal end and low frequency components traveling more slowly to the apical end. For sufficiently small frequencies, those below about 40 Hz, there is no peak, just a gradual increase in amplitude, and the apical end of the basilar membrane simply "wags" up and down at the impressed frequency. Possibly at these low frequencies the hair cells send pulses of electrical energy that the brain can "count" to determine the pitch. If so, a volley theory applies for these very low frequencies. The helicotrema may play a role at these frequencies, with the fluid in the scala vestibuli able to push through it into and out of the scala tympani.

The evolution of the ear has involved interesting compromises among the various competing factors in order to provide an efficient hearing mechanism. There is remarkably little friction in the operation of

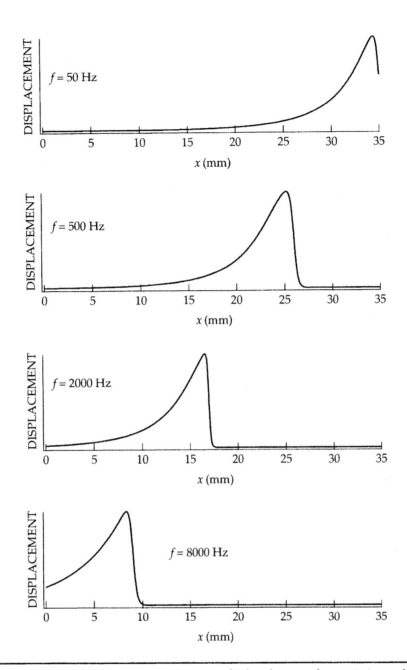

FIGURE 12-11   Schematic diagram of wave envelopes on the basilar membrane as input frequency changes.

the ear despite the fact that fluids are present. With low friction, one could conceive of a uniform basilar membrane on which waves traveled to the apex, reflected back, and formed standing waves. In this case, the ear would be most sensitive to the resonant frequencies of the basilar membrane and not so much to the frequencies in between these. That would be unsatisfactory, of course. Thus, having different portions of the basilar membrane sensitive to different fre-

quencies is a superior mechanism. That requires the properties of the membrane to vary as one proceeds from one end to the other; but if there were sudden changes in properties, one would expect reflections, as we have discussed in terms of impedance mismatches. In the case of the basilar membrane, the changes take place gradually enough that reflections are negligible.

While the traveling wave theory is widely

accepted, there are certainly aspects of the hearing process that seem to require further refinements of the theory. Correspondingly, further experimental progress needs to be made to clarify many issues. The peaks, as found by Békésy, analogous to those shown schematically in Figure 12-11, were too broad to explain the ear's frequency discrimination as shown in psychoacoustic experiments and by neural responses (such as the sensitivity of 2 or 3 Hz around 1000 Hz mentioned above). However, Békésy did his research on dead subjects and with high-amplitude inputs to the inner ear. More recent experiments, on live subjects and at much lower input amplitudes, have demonstrated a much closer correspondence experimentally between the frequency selectivity of the basilar membrane and that of the neural responses.

A traveling wave theory based simply on the mechanical properties (elasticity, density, etc.) of the basilar membrane and surrounding fluid is apparently unable to account for all the features now experimentally found, including the frequency sensitivity of the ear. This is perhaps to be expected, since the living ear contains electrical processes in the hair cells and nerves that do not occur in dead ears, and a simple mechanical model excludes these processes. In a live ear, the electrical activity could play a role in sharpening the mechanical discrimination of the basilar membrane. Further, recent experiments on live ears have shown that the ear is a nonlinear device, and this was not a feature of the strictly mechanical theories. While the field of nonlinear systems is very complicated and is still the subject of active biological research, we can mention a few points.

A spring is a linear device: if we double the force on it, the distance it stretches is doubled. But devices exist that behave quite differently, so that each doubling of the force causes, say, four times the stretch. Such a device is **nonlinear**. If we make a medium out of a nonlinear elastic material and send waves onto it, we will find some interesting things. Suppose we send in a complex input wave initially made up of two sinusoidal waves of frequency f_1 and f_2. We would find that a resulting complex wave on the nonlinear material contains not only our original frequency components f_1 and f_2, but also waves having frequencies that are sums and differences of the original two frequencies, such as, $f_1 + f_2$ and $f_1 - f_2$, and $2f_1 - f_2$. Such waves are called **combination tones**. The interesting thing is we do indeed hear such tones. In the acoustic experiment, two pure tones are played, and the listener hears both those tones and the combination tones. The latter components do not actually exist in the sound wave entering the ear; the ear creates these

new tones on it own. This result is certain evidence that the ear's detection system is nonlinear.

In some nonlinearities, the response of the medium depends on how big the response itself is. That strange situation is best explained by the common example of an amplifier **feedback loop**. When a speaker using an amplifier carries the microphone too close to a loudspeaker, or when the volume is turned up too high, the loudspeaker emits a squeal. The speaker uses the microphone to amplify her voice; the microphone picks up the louder sound from the loudspeaker and feeds it back to the amplifier, which reamplifies it again, which the microphone again picks up, and so on. Of course, the amplifier cannot provide an infinitely loud sound, so it soon saturates at the loud squeal of a **feedback oscillation**.

A somewhat similar feedback process might occur in the ear, in which the position of the largest-amplitude traveling wave excites hair cells, and the electrical activity at that point selectively amplifies the displacement of that point to further excite the electrical mechanism. This would result in enhanced frequency discrimination. Electrical activity of the hair cells is certainly caused by the mechanical motion of the basilar membrane; the suggestion here is that the opposite is also possible, namely, that electrical hair cell activity can cause mechanical response of the basilar membrane. The latter would cause motion of the stapes and the eardrum, finally resulting in sound emanating from the ear. Such **otoacoustic emissions** have been detected, either accompanying stimulation of the ear by external sounds, or in some cases from an ear having no stimulation at all. Such emissions can be used to detect hearing pathologies.

The exact mechanism by which the ear does frequency discrimination, nonlinear behavior, and many related matters are still the subject of intensive research.

12-D. *The Process of Hearing*

As a summary of the hearing mechanism, we trace a sound signal through the entire system.

a) Sound wave (pressure fluctuations) enters the ear canal.

b) Pressure fluctuations cause the eardrum to vibrate. These are mechanical vibrations not unlike the vibrations of a drum head.

c) Vibrations of the eardrum are transmitted to the ossicles via the malleus.

d) The malleus transmits vibrations to the stapes via lever action. The stapes pivots, thereby oscillating the oval window.

e) Motions of the oval window cause the fluid in the cochlea to move.

f) The fluid motions cause pressure variations along the cochlear partition and, in particular, cause traveling wave vibrations to proceed along the basilar membrane.

g) Motions of the basilar membrane cause relative motion of the Organ of Corti and the bending of hairs cells.

h) Hair cell motions trigger nerve cells, causing electrical signals to be sent to the brain.

At the threshold of hearing, the eardrum's amplitude of oscillations is about 10^{-11} m. That's a really tiny amount of movement. (The diameter of a hydrogen atom is about 10^{-11} m.) The amplitude of oscillations of the basilar membrane are even smaller than that of the eardrum. The ear is sensitive to intensities ranging over 12 orders of magnitude. It is an amazing instrument.

Exercises

1. A lever is used to lift a 20 N weight by use of a 2 N force. The short lever arm is 3 m long. How long is the long lever arm?

2. The middle ear carries out its function of getting sound energy from air into the liquid of the inner ear *mainly* by

   a) diffraction.

   b) concentrating the force on the eardrum onto the smaller area of the oval window.

   c) acting as a lever.

   d) increasing the amount of sound reflected at the eardrum.

   e) setting up standing waves between the eardrum and the oval window.

3. Suppose the ear canal were 2 inches long. What effect would that have on hearing sensitivity?

4. A car jack allows one to lift a portion of a car, weighing 1000 lbs, off the ground by application of a force of just 5 lbs. What is the amplification factor of the jack? Explain how this makes sense in terms of the work input by the operator to the jack and work done by the jack on the car? Is there a distance difference, as in the lever?

5. Suppose the short arm on a lever is 0.2 m and the long arm is 2 m. How much weight can one lift with the application of 10 N of force?

6. If a sound wave is proceeding from water into air (the opposite of the example considered in the text), what percentage of the intensity would be transmitted?

7. The ratio of impedances of two substances is $R = 5$. What percentage of intensity is reflected at the boundary?

8. Suppose that the cochlea were a nearly friction-free uniform sheet 35 mm long with all waves traveling at 35 m/s. To what frequencies would the ear be most sensitive? Use a model of a string of that length tied at both ends. Would such an hearing mechanism be described under the classification of a place theory, a temporal theory, or neither?

9. If someone were discovered to have approximately a 30 dB hearing loss across all frequencies, what would a likely diagnosis be for that person's problem?

10. Helmholtz is said to have described the ear by analogy with a harp. Explain in what ways that might be a good or a bad analogy.

11. A carpenter hits a nail with a 50 N force. The area of the nail head is $2.5 \times 10^{-5}\,m^2$, while the point of the nail is $2.5 \times 10^{-7}m^2$. What pressure is applied by the nail point?

A
Metric System of Units

The metric measurement scheme, known as the International System of Units or, simply, SI units after the French Le Système International d'Unites, is based on the meter, second, and kilogram as the basic measures of length, time, and mass, respectively. We will not go into the details of how one sets the standards of each of these quantities, but rather simply give approximate equivalencies of various metric quantities to their more familiar English counterparts.

For example, a length of 1 meter (m) is approximately 39.4 inches or 3.28 feet (a bit longer than an yardstick). There are 100 centimeters (cm) and 1000 millimeters (mm) in 1 m, so 1 cm = 0.394 inches, or 2.54 cm per inch. A kilometer is 1000 m, which equals 0.6 miles.

Mass is related to the amount of material in a body and is not equivalent to weight. Weight is the amount of pull of gravity on a body. This force depends on the mass but would differ whether the mass is on Earth or, say, on the moon, which pulls on a body with 1/6 Earth's force of gravity. Mass is measured in kilograms (kg), whereas force is measured in newtons (N). The English unit of force is the pound. The English unit of mass is unfamiliar to most people, and we do not even bother to introduce it. However, we can relate the SI unit of mass to its weight on Earth; a 1 kg mass would weigh 2.2 pounds on Earth.

The following table gives the equivalencies for length, mass, force, velocity, and pressure. Other SI units, such as energy, power, and intensity, are introduced in detail in the text as we need them.

Note also the following SI prefixes: kilo- = 10^3, centi- = 10^{-2}, milli- = 10^{-3} as in 1 kilometer (km) = 10^3 m = 1000 m, 1 centimeter (cm) = 0.01 m, and 1 millisecond (ms) = 0.001 s.

TABLE A-1   SI Units and Their Equivalent English Units.

Quantity	Metric Unit	English Equivalent
Length	1 meter (m)	39.4 inches (in) = 3.28 feet (ft)
	1 kilometer (km)	0.62 mile (mi)
Time	1 second (s)	1 second
Mass	1 kilogram (kg)	2.2 pounds (lbs) weight on Earth
Velocity	1 meter per second (m/s)*	3.28 feet per second (ft/s)
	1 kilometer per hour (km/hr)	0.62 mph
Force	1 newton (N)†	0.225 lbs
Pressure	1 Pascal (Pa or N/m²)‡	1.45×10^{-4} pounds per in² (psi)

*speed of sound in air = 335 m/s = 750 mph = 1100 ft/s
†1 kg weighs 9.8 N.
‡ atmospheric pressure is 14.7 psi = 1.013×10^5 Pa

B
Phonetic Symbols Used

Here we provide a listing of the symbols used to indicate sounds in spoken language. The standard method of writing English (and many other languages) is called orthography. However, in the standard correct spelling of words, the same symbol is often used to indicate many different pronunciations. For example, [g] as in "go," [dʒ] as in "George," and [ʒ] as in "rouge" are all spelled with the letter "g" in English. For that reason, phonetic symbols have been developed to give an accurate printed representation of spoken sounds.

The worldwide standard is the International Phonetic Alphabet (IPA). In IPA, each sound must be represented by a different symbol. Shown in Table B-1 are orthographic symbols for some of the sounds in English, the corresponding IPA symbols, and words to illustrate the corresponding sounds. We do not include symbols for consonants that represent the same sound as the corresponding English letters: [p], [b], [t], [d], [k], [m], [n], [f], [v], [s], [z], [l], [w]; e.g., [t] in "tea."

For further information, consult the International Phonetic Association's *Handbook* (International Phonetic Association 1999) or Web site at *http://www2. arts.gla.ac.uk/IPA/ipa.html*.

TABLE B-1 Orthographic Symbols, IPA Symbols, and Words Illustrating the Sounds

Consonants		
Orthographic Symbol	**IPA Symbol**	**Key Word**
g	g	**g**o
ng	ŋ	ri**ng**
y	j	**y**ou
r	ɹ	**r**ed
th	θ	**th**igh
th	ð	**th**y
sh	ʃ	**sh**oe
g	ʒ	rou**g**e
ch	tʃ	**ch**urch
j, g	dʒ	**j**u**dg**e
(glottal stop)	ʔ	**uh-oh**

(continues)

TABLE B-1   *Continued*

Vowels		
Orthographic Symbol	**IPA Symbol**	**Key Word**
ee, ea, ie, y	i	seed
i	ɪ	sit
a, ay, ai, a_e,* ey	e	say
e	ɛ	sled
a	æ	sad
u, ue, oo, u_e,* ew	u	sue
oo	ʊ	soot
o, oa, o_e,* ough, ow	o	soak
aw, au, augh, ough	ɔ	slaw
o	ɑ	stop
u	ʌ	supper
any vowel letter	ə	about
ir, ur	ɝ	sturdy
er	ɚ	sputter
ow, ough, au, ou	aʊ	spout
i, i_e,* y, uy, igh	aɪ	sigh
oi, oy	ɔɪ	soy

*The underline between two letters stands for any consonant—e.g., "a_e" might mean "ate."

International Phonetic Association (1999). *Handbook of the International Phonetic Association*. Cambridge, UK: Cambridge University Press.

Index

Vocal cords, 97
Vocal folds, 56, 97, 99
Vocal organs, 97
Vocal tract, 56, 87, 97
  acoustical properties, 101–104
  as filter, 87
Voice bar, 142
Voice, 56, 72, 87
  onset time, 146
Voiced consonants, 132, 142, 146
Voicing, 105, 132, 142, 146
Volley theory of hearing, 207
Volume mass density, 15
von Békésy, 207
von Helmholtz, 206
Vowels, 72, 129
  corner, 129
  pure, 129
  schwa, 101, 103
  symbols for, 217
  voiced, 105

Water wave experiment, 2
Watt per square meter, 185
Watt, 177
Wave, 1
  antisymmetric, 80
  complex, 65–73, 100
  definition of, 2
  displacement, 41, 45
  energy, 59, 173–176
    and amplitude, 59, 175
  front, 59–63
  glottal, 97, 99–101

impulsive, 5
longitudinal, 2
of mixed symmetry, 80
one-dimensional, 59
oscillatory, 5
plane, 62
pressure, 41, 45
reflection of, 16
repeating, 5, 99
shape, 5
sinusoidal, 2
sound, 1
standing, 5, 27, 209
symmetric, 79
three-dimensional, 60
transmission of, 16
transverse, 2
traveling wave theory of hearing, 207–210
traveling, 5
two-dimensional, 59
velocity, 5
  and f and λ, 11
  and properties of medium, 13–15
Wavelength, 6, 8
  and f and v, 11–12
  allowed, 31, 34, 36, 47
Weight, 13, 171, 215
Whisper, 107, 142
White noise, 73
  on a spectrogram, 105
Wide band spectrogram, 105
Work, 169
  negative, 172
  work-energy theorem, 170, 172

Fundamentals of Sound with Applications to Speech and Hearing